Let us be keen, and rather cut a little,
Than fall and bruise to death.
Shakespeare

The Decision: Your prostate biopsy shows cancer. Now what?

Medical insight, personal stories, and humor by a urologist who has been where you are now.

John C. McHugh M.D.

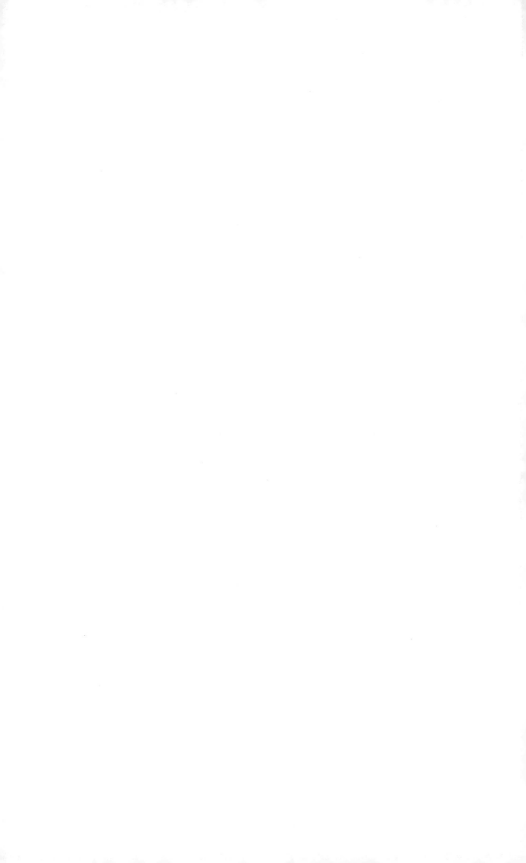

theprostatedecision.com
Theprostatedecision.wordpress.com

Follow Dr. McHugh at http://twitter.com/prostatediaries

Wholesale orders are available at theprostatedecision.com.

The Decision: Your prostate biopsy shows cancer. Now what?

ISBN 978-0-692-00565-1

Editing:

    Johanna Craig Ph.D.

    Sandra Brim Ph.D.

    Janice K. Watts

Cover design and photography:

    Travis Massey

Illustrations:

    Graham Gaines

    Will Black

Formatting/Layout:

    Keith McLeod

Special thanks:

    The staff of Northeast Georgia Urologic Associates for their help in making the unfinished manuscript available to patients over the course of the last year, and their willingness to listen to the author talk about "my book" ad nauseam.

Some of the anecdotal illustrations in this book are true to life and are included with the permission of the persons involved. All other illustrations are composites of real situations, and any resemblance to people living or dead is coincidental.

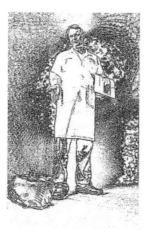

Jennie Cooper Press
"Calm as a hurricane"

To the strong women who have been so important to me throughout my life: Bessie Clay Morgan Davis, Jennie Cooper Davis McHugh, and, most importantly, my wife, Karen. Karen was so beautifully strong throughout my cancer journey, not only for me, but in the navigation of "my predicament," for our children. For that, and for so many things, I am forever grateful and in her debt.

The newly diagnosed patient with prostate cancer, too, will learn of the prominent role the women in his life will play in his journey. Trust me.

TABLE OF CONTENTS

Bias - *Do you have a dog in this fight?*

Cure-driven - *Most aggressive treatment is your priority.*

Risk-driven - *Least chance of side effects is your priority.*

Lifestyle-driven - *Ease of treatment is your priority.*

Internet/family/friends - *Apples to apples/Prostates to prostates.*

Misconceptions and half-truths - *Don't let "a little knowledge" get you.*

McHugh Decision Worksheet - *Have you learned enough about yourself and your prostate cancer to answer these questions intelligently?*

Getting your priorities straight - *Paper covers rock.*

You've got good health and all options are open to you - *Evaluating your underlying health is an important part of the decision process.*

Evaluating the negatives - *Picking your poison.*

Best case/worse case scenarios - *Evaluating the potential outcome of your decision from different perspectives may be of help to you.*

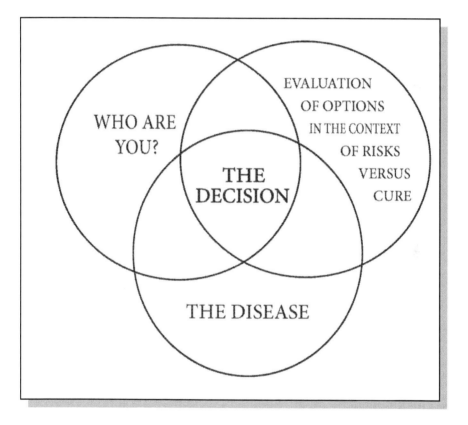

Introduction-Now you know and the process begins

*Y*ou've just experienced the anxiety, humiliation and pain of having your prostate biopsied. Since the biopsy you have endured the sight of blood in your urine and bowel movements, blood in your semen, and burning when you void. You have been told that the bleeding is to be expected, but to notify the doctor if you have fever or difficulty voiding. If you have been sexually active, the blood that you and your wife saw was much more than you expected when the doctor warned you of this possibility. You wonder if you have hurt something or if somehow the blood in your semen could transfer anything to your wife. You wished you had asked that question. Now you begin to ponder the possible outcome of the biopsy and whether it will be positive, and you feel a wave of intense anxiety churn across your chest. Although your wife loves you and wants to help, you suffer this "waiting time" silently and alone. Thoughts of the negative possibilities and how each could impact the people you love, your work, and your longevity run rampant in your mind throughout the day and week. In an odd way you feel as though you have let your family down just by being in this situation. Your anxiety increases as the day approaches for the follow-up office visit to learn of the biopsy results; the butterflies return and become more frequent and intense. You begin to think, "The doctor would have called by now if the results were good," and this suspicion adds to the tension. Your normal daily activities, work, going to church, playing tennis, whatever, feel surreal with the result of the biopsy and its attendant ramifications looming over you. The days pass with the incessant mental examination of all the potential possibilities. Thoughts like "what will I do if it's positive" abound, but life goes on. You pay bills, deal with your children, and handle other problems as if nothing else were going *on with your health. That is all you can do. You now glaringly understand the truism that life does indeed go on, and finally you transition into an attitude of acceptance: "what will be, will be." This newfound attitude of relinquishing control over life and the results of your biopsy is, in a sense, a resignation, but it is comforting. Your preacher's admonitions to "Give it over to God" ring clear to you now and have relevance to you as never before. On the day of the doctor's appointment to receive the results, you leave work early, and the butterflies reappear yet again. They multiply in waves in the waiting room, reaching an uninterrupted crescendo as your name is called and you are escorted to your chair in the exam room. There you wait; your heart pounding so loudly you feel those outside the room must hear it. Your thoughts turn again to the what-ifs: to your children, your wife, or someone you know who died of prostate cancer. You wonder if your affairs are in order and how your parents would feel about having a son with cancer. The doorknob turns, startling you, and the door opens. You attempt in vain to read the expression on the doctor's face, looking for signs of good news, but you realize that the doctor's face portends the news you hoped you would not hear: "I am sorry; I have bad news for you. Your prostate biopsy shows cancer."*

An arrow in your quiver

W hat is it that this book hopes to achieve, and why was it written? The aim of this book is to systematically break down the issues that are necessary for you to come to a decision as to what form of treatment, if any, you want to pursue. At the moment a patient is told he has prostate cancer, he and his family become thirsty for knowledge about the cancer and what should be done to treat it. After an overview of the options to the extent an office visit will allow, I usually refer my patients to sites on the Internet and give them a book on the subject given to me for free by a drug company. These books explain the disease and nicely lay out the available treatment options, but they do not provide a method to personalize the decision-making process to achieve the most appropriate treatment for you. What the patient assumed was a straightforward, non-fatal disease of old men becomes, after research, much more complicated and potentially fatal.

Patients are often frustrated when making the decision about how to proceed with treatment because there are so many variables in terms of options and associated risks. I diagnosed a friend of mine, a surgeon, and shortly thereafter he showed up at my home with a bottle of wine and a legal pad with three pages of questions. "I had no idea how complicated this disease and the treatment of it were, John." In over 20 years of practicing urology, I have seen this scenario played out many times. Books available on prostate cancer are myriad in number and scope, but I feel they do not focus on the issue at hand: "the decision" and how to make it.

Right now, you don't need a big, comprehensive book about the causes and intricacies of prostate cancer; that is irrelevant to you.

In making your decision about how to treat it, you need to know what is important and relevant *in your circumstances*. This book combines the professional and personal experience of a surgeon who has treated hundreds of patients with prostate cancer and has also been through the agonizing decision-making process and treatment himself. In addition, I have added personal, sometimes humorous, stories of my journey that I hope will add some reality and texture to your understanding of this disease and what you might experience, which in turn may aid you in your decision.

Another novel facet of this book is that it highlights the significance of considering different therapies' effects on the male voiding pattern. As a urologist, I cannot emphasize enough the importance you should place on how you void, or as my attending physician during my urologic residency called it, "make your water." How you void and how you will void after treatment is, I feel, a very important and an often overlooked factor in the decision-making process. I will make clear the effects of the various treatment methods on how you void, and I will stress why it is so important to weigh this aspect of the decision in its rightful perspective. I offer to you my years of experience in diagnosing this disease, treating this disease, and having this disease as tools in choosing the right treatment for you. This book is not a reference book on prostate cancer; there are many books and sources available for that. There are no footnotes; all that is written is from my personal experience, both in dealing with my cancer and in helping my patients through the process as well. It is, however, a necessary "arrow in your quiver" to be used *in addition* to your other resources in the journey to making an appropriate "decision."

Preface

The urologist I chose to do my surgery I had never met, spoken to, or recommended to anyone. At my initial appointment, his nurse escorted me to his office, where he was waiting. After we shook hands and introduced ourselves, there was a somewhat uncomfortable pause, with the two of us sitting across from each other in silence. It was odd, two urologists who had never met, one needing surgery for something that both were accustomed to treating. "So, doctor…" he said, "you have your own disease."

> It's not the mountains ahead, but the pebbles in your shoes.

I was diagnosed with prostate cancer at the age of 52. I believe I was lucky in that it was detected early and treated aggressively without any major complications, and hopefully I am done with it. I owe my personal diligence in diagnosing my cancer early, in part, to the knowledge of a friend whose father, Dr. Cecil L. Miller of Buford, Georgia, died of prostate cancer. In fact, I called Butch shortly after my diagnosis not to tell him about me, but to be sure he had had a recent rectal exam and PSA. He asked why I had thought to call him, and I told him, "I will tell you another time; something interesting happened to me that made me think of you." Butch's father was a family physician whose first symptom of prostate cancer was bone pain, indicating that his prostate cancer, which was unknown to him, had spread to bone. He was diagnosed at age 72 in September; he died the following June. My friend's father's story has had a lasting impact on me. Certainly the fact that this man was a doctor, experiencing no symptoms, and diagnosed with metastatic prostate cancer when it was too late to treat it was a tragic event. It made me more aware of the potentially virulent side of what is usually thought of as a "slow-growing" cancer. His story made me more vigilant about advising my patients about the dual nature of prostate cancer and making sure I checked up on my prostate. I began having PSAs at age 48 and watched as they slowly increased from the normal range to abnormal over four years. This led to the biopsy, the diagnosis, and, finally, the treatment. It took me three months to decide which mode of treatment I would choose. The anguish experienced in determining which form of therapy to pursue, something I had witnessed over the years in hundreds of my patients, was now perpetrated upon me.

For reasons I hope to make clear to you, the decision, though a difficult one to make if all relevant factors are taken into account, can be simplified by using big concepts. This book is written primarily for the patient with newly diagnosed prostate cancer, as an aid in arriving at a treatment decision that is right for him, and, more importantly, made for the right reason. Nothing is as disappointing as the patient who bases his choice on incorrect or irrelevant information and subsequently has an unexpected, sub-optimal outcome. I am a surgeon, so feel free to take what I say with a grain of salt. I do favor the surgical removal of the prostate in general, but only in the right circumstances, with the patient having full knowledge of the ramifications of all therapeutic modalities. The decision is always the patient's to make, and it's a tough one. My goal is to give you the knowledge of what is essential to know about prostate cancer, taken in the context of your particular situation, and to aid you in making an intelligent decision custom-made for you.

I hope that my journey to "the decision" and my many years of helping others through it will be beneficial to you. By reading this book you become privy to information you might get in an extended office visit with your own personal board-certified urologist. The illustrations that follow are based on sketches I have drawn many times on exam table paper for my own patients, and they are intended to simplify concepts patients need to understand when considering treatment options. *In addition, I offer the perspective of a urologist who has been through what you are about to experience.* Despite my years of training and experience, my decision was based on big concepts rather than the fine points of various treatments or their potential for particular risks. As you go through this process, you too should use big concepts to make your decision and not be bogged down by "the pebbles in your shoes."

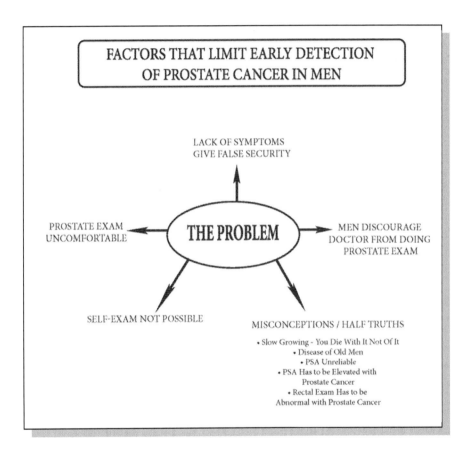

Part One – The basics

Prostate cancer and the male - *The perfect storm*

A little knowledge is a dangerous thing.

My mother loved to use old adages as aids to imparting advice as life's learning experiences arose. Although "the pot calling the kettle black," "it's going to be too wet to plough," and "you can lead a horse to water but you can't make him drink," were commonly called upon, I believe "a little knowledge is a dangerous thing" was her favorite. She reminded me of the saying so many times that as I got older, she only needed to say, "a little knowledge John" with a sarcastic upward inflection in her voice, and I knew what she meant. In no other disease does this saying ring so true as in prostate cancer and men's perception of it.

Most men know very little about the prostate in terms of what it does, what it looks like, or where it is located in their body. Upon telling my little brother Jeff, who was 46 at the time, that I had prostate cancer, he asked, "Is the prostate like that little tube you took out when you did my vasectomy?" What little men do know or have heard about the prostate is often either incorrect or only partially true. This is where a little knowledge can be a very dangerous thing. Most patients know just enough about the prostate to hurt them. This is true of both the patient who does not have prostate cancer and the one who has researched the disease after his diagnosis. "Most people die with it, instead of because of it" and "It's a disease of old men," are common misconceptions prevalent among patients. Although these concepts have some degree of truth, the problem is in the word "most." It is this thinking that lowers men's diligence for early detection, and after diagnosis they make decisions based on these partially true perceptions.

The fact is that more than 200,000 men per year are diagnosed with prostate cancer, and each year almost 25,000 men die of it. Fifty-year-old men and younger are commonly diagnosed with prostate cancer, often the more aggressive form. The perception that prostate cancer does not kill or is only a concern for the elderly is wrong and hampers men from making a point to be examined. Unlike the breast in a female, the prostate in a male is not amenable to a self-exam. Men also believe, incorrectly, that prostate cancer causes voiding symptoms, and they assume that if they have no symptoms, there is no need to be checked. This too is an impediment to early diagnosis. Most prostate cancers occur well away from the channel in the prostate that men urinate through, so in early prostate cancer, voiding is normal. Symptoms occur late in prostate cancer and are usually indicative of advanced disease. If a man waits until he has symptoms to be checked, he has waited too long. Despite this, men I see frequently tell me that they don't want to have a rectal exam because they have no voiding symptoms.

In addition to all of these factors that delay early detection, the necessity of a rectal exam further complicates the situation. The patient often finds ways to avoid having a rectal exam because it is unpleasant, uncomfortable, and, for many men, embarrassing. It is not unusual for patients to suggest, and I am sure that this is the case with many primary care providers as well, "let's do that next time" in response to the suggestion of a prostate exam. Both the patient and the physician, through better education, need to do a better job of making sure rectal exams are done; "out of sight, out of mind" cannot rule the day in this regard. **So the perfect storm: common misconceptions that give men a false sense of security, an exam they do not want to have done, and the resultant flawed rationalization to skip a prostate evaluation. All of these factors contribute to missed opportunities for early detection.**

Although you would have been better off to have had a negative biopsy, the good news for the reader is that you have overcome the previously mentioned hurdles, had the rectal exam and biopsy, and now you know your diagnosis. You have to know that you have prostate cancer in order to treat it. The primary focus of this book is to help guide you through the process to arrive at a decision that is best suited to you. A secondary goal is that, with your new-found knowledge about prostate cancer, the pitfalls related to men's health, and the importance of early diagnosis, you will be proactive in educating others. My hope is that this book will help you with the issues that you are now facing, and aid in preventing the "a little knowledge is a dangerous thing" mentality from precluding early detection in other men.

The PSA, rectal exam, and biopsy report - *The "big three" are the essence of prostate cancer and define the aggressiveness of the disease. An understanding of each is imperative to "The Decision."*

PSA (Prostate Specific Antigen) - *An elevated PSA doesn't mean you have prostate cancer, just that you need to be checked for it.*

The prostate specific antigen (PSA) test is often the first indicator of prostate cancer. Very much like prostate cancer itself, many aspects of the value of the PSA test are poorly understood. PSA is an enzyme normally produced by the prostate. When it was discovered that prostate cancer cells produce more PSA than normal prostate cells, it began to be used as a marker for prostate cancer. Although an elevated PSA can be an early manifestation of prostate cancer, it can be elevated for many other reasons as well. Sex the night before blood is drawn for the test, a recent prostate infection, an enlarged prostate, and a variation or error in the lab testing can all account for an abnormal value. As a result, only about 15% of all patients referred to a urologist for a prostate biopsy on the basis of an elevated PSA result receive a positive diagnosis of prostate cancer. This leads many to proclaim that the test is flawed and results in too many unnecessary biopsies. It seems almost daily that a patient will ask me about the validity of the PSA because of an article in the paper or something they've read on the internet questioning the clinical usefulness of this test.

If your PSA is elevated and you have had a biopsy that was negative, this is great on two fronts. First of all, the biopsy did not reveal cancer. Secondly and more importantly, it pretty much rules out the potential of ever having the bad kind of prostate cancer. You may still be evaluated with serial PSAs and maybe even have a second or third biopsy because of your elevated PSA at some point in the future, but you are essentially off the hook for the kind of prostate cancer that kills quickly. If cancer is ever found on a subsequent biopsy of your prostate, it will most likely be the slow-growing type.

Some may agree that doing biopsies on all patients with elevated PSA is not cost effective, but no one would disagree that measuring PSA as a marker for prostate cancer has saved lives. I can recount many times in when a patient with no symptoms and a normal prostate gland on exam has been found to have significant disease after a biopsy prompted by an abnormal PSA. I have a particular patient in mind who was 39 years old and had the PSA test only because it was part of a panel of tests required for a job physical. His high PSA set in motion a referral to me, a biopsy, and ultimately a diagnosis of prostate cancer. This was an interesting and fortunate situation because a patient this age would not normally have a PSA done. The PSA clearly aided in the diagnosis and probably saved a life. The PSA is a tool that is utilized by the physician in guiding recommendations. It is not a perfect marker for prostate cancer, but it is very helpful.

A fool with a tool is still a fool.

Many patients request only the PSA, thinking that if this value is normal, then a rectal is not necessary and that one probably doesn't have prostate cancer. The reason this happens often is that adding the PSA to blood work already ordered is easy to do; but having the rectal exam done to you is not. The notion that a normal PSA can alone determine if you have prostate cancer is erroneous; it is only a tool to be used with other information about you in deciding whether to proceed to a prostate biopsy. It is not uncommon to have a normal PSA and still have prostate cancer.

The pitfalls of the PSA aside, it also can help in determining the aggressiveness of your disease and deciding how to proceed with treatment. A PSA value is considered elevated if it is over 4. Moderately elevated values range from 4 to 10. If your PSA is over 10, then knowledge of this in addition to the rectal exam and the path report specifics may incline you to take a more aggressive approach to treatment. If you choose surgery, the PSA, rectal exam, and path report can offer guidance as to the potential for the disease extending to the prostate capsule, the membrane covering the prostate, and hence requiring post-surgical radiation. If you are inclined toward radiation, the above information may offer guidance regarding the need for combination radiation therapy, which combines the placement of radioactive seeds inside the capsule (to treat the cancer in the prostate) and external radiation (to treat any disease that may be in the capsule itself).

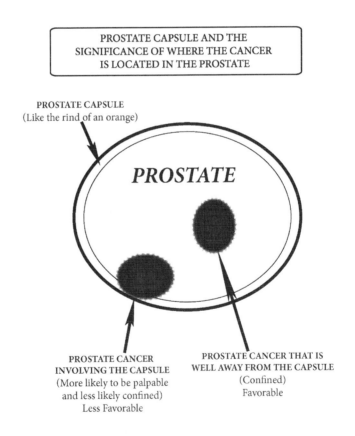

PROSTATE CAPSULE AND THE
SIGNIFICANCE OF WHERE THE CANCER
IS LOCATED IN THE PROSTATE

PROSTATE CAPSULE
(Like the rind of an orange)

PROSTATE

PROSTATE CANCER
INVOLVING THE CAPSULE
(More likely to be palpable
and less likely confined)
Less Favorable

PROSTATE CANCER THAT IS
WELL AWAY FROM THE CAPSULE
(Confined)
Favorable

The rectal exam - *The male patient doesn't want it done and the doctor is easily persuaded not to do it.*

This may sound odd to you, but sometimes you have to demand that a rectal exam be performed. A nurse that I work with in the operating room related to me that her husband, who is in his early 40s, was scheduled for a yearly company physical. She told him to be sure to have a rectal exam and a PSA test, but when he asked his doctor, he was told, "You are too young to have prostate cancer." Upon hearing what transpired, his wife, my co-worker, said, "You go get you another doctor that will do that exam; I work with a bunch of urologists and I know what can happen with prostate cancer!"

An easy way to get a rectal exam and PSA done is to look for free prostate screenings during Prostate Cancer Awareness Month. My community has one every year, and it is an easy way to get checked at a convenient time and at no expense. Usually the urologists will do the rectal exams, and the hospital arranges with a lab company to do the PSA. One year I was doing the rectal exams in the hospital for one such screening and saw a friend of mine, a plastic surgeon, walking down the hall toward me. He was cutting through this area of the hospital to get somewhere else and had just happened upon me. "What are you doing, John?" "I am doing rectal exams for the hospital's prostate screening promotion." This physician has subsequently passed away, and I think of him often and his fun-loving spirit. "Can I have one?" "Well sure. Now?" "Yes, if it is O.K.?" At that point, hardly even breaking stride, he detoured into the room off the hall and all in one swoop flipped up his lab coat, dropped his pants, and said," I'm ready!" I checked the prostate, and told him it was normal. He pulled up his pants, flipped down his lab coat, thanked me, and then, just as quickly as he had come, went on his way. I mention this story to make the point that when it comes to a rectal exam, you've got to get one when you can.

When I began my practice in Urology in 1986, a biopsy of the prostate was recommended if there was a palpable abnormality on rectal exam. All men, then as now, were advised to have a rectal exam yearly, usually beginning at the age of 50. If an abnormality was found, the prostate biopsy was usually performed at the hospital under anesthesia, as it was very painful. The biopsies performed were limited in number and to the area of the abnormality, usually a palpable nodule. The biopsy device was placed on the nodule with the exam finger and done blindly, in other words guided by the urologist's finger by feel. (The fear of the needle hitting your finger by accident was so great, as urologic residents we would joke about the pathology report coming back "normal finger.") The blood test that was used at the time, Prostatic acid phosphatase, was usually obtained, but this was only indicative of prostate cancer metastasis, not the diagnosis of prostate cancer.

Today the most common reason for a biopsy of the prostate is an elevated PSA, not a palpable abnormality. In fact, if a patient presents today with a palpable nodule, it usually represents a cancer that is further advanced than is desirable. Biopsies of the prostate are now done with the aid of a rectal ultrasound probe that guides the biopsy device to the desired location. Most urologists do about 12 biopsies in a specified pattern to sample the entire prostate. Having a normal prostate exam is a great start but does not get you off the hook regarding the need for a biopsy or whether you have cancer or not. If the gland is normal to exam but the PSA is high, you still need a biopsy. I have seen on many occasions a normal prostate exam associated with a minimally elevated PSA, and all the biopsies revealing prostate cancer.

Shortly after turning 50 I arranged with a friend of mine, who is a gastroenterologist, to have a routine colonoscopy done. When I went for my initial visit, my friend asked me a number of questions about my medical history, examined my heart and abdomen, and then told me what to expect with the colonoscopy. After I left, I realized that I had forgotten to ask him to examine my prostate and neither did he offer to do a prostate exam. I had been monitoring my PSA, and it was closing in on abnormal. I wanted to be sure there was not a palpable issue with my prostate. I was well aware that one can have a grossly abnormal prostate upon exam in spite of having a normal or slightly abnormal PSA, and I had not had a rectal exam since medical school. (It had been performed on me by a fellow female medical student twenty years previously as part of an introductory class on physical exams. I distinctly remember not having had the opportunity of returning the favor of performing a breast exam on her.) After the colonoscopy, as my friend was leaving, I remembered to ask him to do a rectal exam. He turned back around, examined the prostate, said that both my prostate and colonoscopy were normal, and went on his way. A year or so later in the hospital parking lot I told him that I had had a recent prostate biopsy and had prostate cancer. "What did your rectal show?" he asked immediately. I told him that I had asked my partner do one before my biopsy, and it was also normal. My friend slumped his shoulders with a sigh of relief, as he was concerned that he might have missed a subtle irregularity. I know that feeling. No doctor wants to have missed something early on

*that could have made a difference in a patient's care. This story
again illustrates how the rectal exam is often times pushed to the
side, and that the patient needs to know the importance of it to be
proactive in having it done. A man 45 or older does not leave my
office unless I have an accounting of his last rectal exam and
whether it needs to be done. I go so far as to tell patients," If I
recommend it and you decline it, I will document that in my
dictation." To be a urologist and miss prostate cancer because you
didn't perform a rectal exam would be, as my mother would say,
"a cardinal sin."*

So, how does your rectal exam play into your decision-making
after the diagnosis has been made? If you have been told you have
prostate cancer and your rectal exam before the biopsy was
normal, then your prostate cancer is either very early or of the
infiltrative type. In other words, it is not all in one spot and
forming a palpable nodule. A normal exam often, but not always,
means there is minimal disease and that your cancer has been
detected early. As mentioned, it can be extensive, in an infiltrative
or spreading fashion, and still not be palpable. Having a normal
exam is like having good health when you are beginning the
decision-making process; all the treatment options are open to you.
If you have a palpable nodule or asymmetry, then this does
somewhat drive the decision to a more aggressive treatment. A
patient is more likely to have capsular extension if there is a nodule
or other palpable abnormality. (Remember the prostate is like an
orange, and the capsule is its rind.)

If you feel that surgery is the most aggressive way to treat prostate
cancer, then knowing you have a palpable abnormality may sway
your decision toward surgery. Alternatively, the patient with a

palpable abnormality who is leaning towards radiation will probably be advised to have combination radiation therapy. The radioactive seeds treat the cancer in the meat of the gland (pulp of the orange), and then external beam radiation is added to cover the possibility of capsular extension (the rind of the orange).

Do you know the specifics of your rectal exam? I bet you that if you are over 45 and have recently had a physical, there is a better than 50-50 chance you had either only a PSA or neither a PSA nor rectal exam done. I'll also bet that you did not question this and were glad that a rectal exam wasn't done. Furthermore, I'll bet your wife asked you about it and is more in tune with the need for you to have your prostate examined than you are.

Pathology report specifics - *When it comes to a positive biopsy, the key issues are Gleason's score and volume of disease.*

This Gleason isn't funny.

The morning I got the results of yet another PSA that was creeping up, I stopped one of my partners outside of an exam room and asked him if he would do a biopsy of my prostate at lunch. He agreed, and I told him I'd have my nurse come get him when I was ready. When the morning patients had been seen, I asked my nurse to set up the stuff for a biopsy, and within an hour of deciding to have my prostate biopsied, I find myself in the biopsy room. I pull down my scrubs, get on the table on my left side, assume the fetal position required for the procedure, and tell Tina, "go get Dr. Jones; I'm ready." In one fell swoop I am exposing my naked backside to my nurse and my partner, and, in doing so beginning my journey as a patient. I had had many patients tell me over the years, "I was modest before I became a urology patient," and now I was getting my "education."

I did take an antibiotic to prevent infection, but I did not take anything for pain. My plan was to have the biopsy, go get lunch, and then come back to see my afternoon patients. Dr. Jones obligingly enters the procedure room to perform the biopsy I have requested just minutes before. "What is your PSA, John?" "Five or so. Will you check my prostate before you begin?" "Sure," he says, "It feels normal." He places the ultrasound probe in the rectal area, and there is an abrupt and intense sensation of needing to void. (Pressure on the prostate by the rigid probe irritates the prostatic urethra. The resultant sensation of needing to void is similar to that experienced by patients after radiation.) He then injects an anesthetic into the prostate to deaden the effect of the biopsies but tells me, "I don't see the seminal vesicles very well." What this means is that the medicine he is injecting may not control the pain of the biopsy. That's a luck thing; my anatomy probably didn't lend itself to a good nerve block. However, altered anatomy can also mean changes as a result of cancer, and my mind immediately went wild, wondering, why my seminal vesicles were difficult to see. He began the process of taking the specimens with a biopsy gun that fires a biopsy needle that, in turn, captures the prostate tissue. You hear a click when it fires and then feel a pain that is similar to a bee sting, but a bee sting that is accompanied by an intense burning at the tip of your "you know what." It felt to me as if someone was popping a rubber band at the tip of my "private area" with each biopsy; he did 16. Somewhere in the middle of this ordeal, as I was debating the wisdom of doing this at lunch without the benefit of pain medicine, Dr. Jones says, "John, shared joy-twice joy, shared sorrow-half sorrow." After these obtuse words of wisdom, which I failed to grasp, came another "pop." I propped up on my elbow and looked back at Dr. Jones over my shoulder. "Twice grief, shared what? What in the world is that supposed to mean, Bill?" Tina says quickly, "He says that to everybody having a biopsy." "Well John, you should share things with people. Don't keep things to yourself; it is better to discuss your problems with friends." Tina added, "Dr. McHugh only has one friend, Dr. Tolson." I said, "What do you mean, share with my friends? Share what? I don't have cancer yet. You just got started! Do you see something back there that you don't like?" "No, not really anything bad, just an area that doesn't look right. I'll take just a few more in that area and we'll be done." The biopsies just kept on coming; a click, a pop, the bee sting, the rubber band, and the incessant feeling of needing to urinate. This adventure into being a patient ended after about 20 minutes. I got up, thanked Bill, and then went into the bathroom dripping blood from the front and back. That afternoon, I had to inform two people that their biopsies for prostate cancer were positive, all the while concerned that blood would show through the front of my scrubs. The next phase of my journey as a patient then began: waiting on the results and wondering if I had cancer at all, if I had the good kind, or if I could be the one with the "tiger" variety, (which is how the British describe the aggressive form of prostate cancer). Again, the dual nature of the disease is something that patients often don't realize.

A biopsy of the prostate involves obtaining a representative sampling of 12-16 small cores of tissue; however, it can give you a clue as to the nature of the cancer in the entire gland and help in your decision-making process. The two most important features of a path report showing prostate cancer are the grade, or Gleason's score, and the number and percentage of positive cores, or volume of disease. The Gleason's score is indicative of the potential aggressiveness of your cancer and is determined by a pathologist, who evaluates the two worst areas (highest grades) of your specimen and assigns each area a number between 1 and 5. The most common Gleason's grade found in positive biopsies is 6, or a 3+3, which is referred to as moderate grade. A Gleason's score of 7, which represents a 3+4, or above is considered high-grade prostate cancer. The score is important because the higher the grade, the more aggressive and unpredictable the cancer. In my opinion, a higher grade should make a patient lean toward a more aggressive treatment.

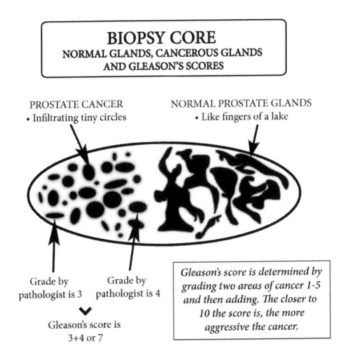

BIOPSY CORE
NORMAL GLANDS, CANCEROUS GLANDS
AND GLEASON'S SCORES

PROSTATE CANCER
• Infiltrating tiny circles

NORMAL PROSTATE GLANDS
• Like fingers of a lake

Grade by pathologist is 3

Grade by pathologist is 4

Gleason's score is 3+4 or 7

Gleason's score is determined by grading two areas of cancer 1-5 and then adding. The closer to 10 the score is, the more aggressive the cancer.

Volume of disease, or percentage of the biopsy cores that contain cancer, particularly if present on both sides of the prostate, is also important as it may indicate the amount of disease in the entire gland. So, low grade and low volume are good things, and high grade and large volume are not as good. Knowing this helps you make a decision regarding your treatment. If you had a choice between having a low grade or low volume, low grade is much better. High grade (Gleason's score 7 or greater) is unpredictable, more aggressive, and accounts for most of the deaths attributed to prostate cancer. If you have a high Gleason's score, you may not have the same results as your friend who had a low Gleason's score and did well with a particular treatment. If you are basing *your* decision on what he did without knowing the specifics of *his* *biopsy*, you are making a decision based on a flawed premise.

PATH REPORT SPECIFICS

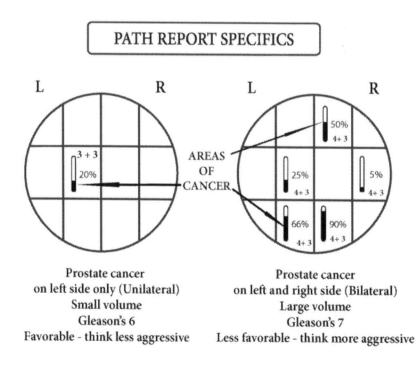

Prostate cancer
on left side only (Unilateral)
Small volume
Gleason's 6
Favorable - think less aggressive

Prostate cancer
on left and right side (Bilateral)
Large volume
Gleason's 7
Less favorable - think more aggressive

One evening I was explaining to my wife a little bit about prostate cancer and the issues she and I faced with the potential ramifications of being treated. When I first told her that the biopsy was positive, she asked, "There's a medicine you can take for that, isn't there?" After educating her about the intricacies of prostate cancer and its treatment, I sought to reassure her that my cancer was found relatively early and that it was likely that my treatment would just be a "major inconvenience."

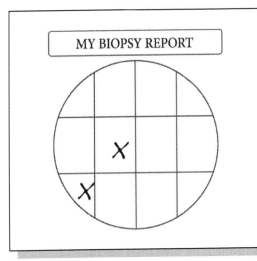

On the back of a paper bag at the kitchen table, I drew a picture of my biopsy report, as seen here, to indicate that only a small amount of cancer had been found and that I should do well with a good chance of cure. I remember being a little emotional talking about it and trying to be up-beat so as not to alarm her. I worried that if she saw my distress, it would cause her to be distressed too. After all, I am the breadwinner, father of our children, and her companion for almost 30 years. As I worried about upsetting her with all this information, she picked up the pencil and began to peer at the diagram I had made. She put another positive area on the picture I had just drawn, then a line through the three areas, and said, "Tic tac toe, John." We stared at her handiwork almost mesmerized, and then she looked up at me and smiled. I thought at the time that I had done a good job of allaying her fears, but in retrospect, maybe she sensed something

in me that prompted her to allay mine. Wives are smart that way.

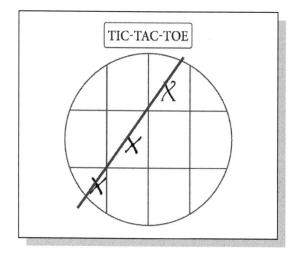

The chart that follows is a simplified overview of the various combinations of Gleason's score and volume of disease seen in prostate biopsies. What I hope you will learn to do is to take each of the issues related to you and your cancer and, for each, evaluate which treatment is best suited to you. As it applies to Gleason's score and volume of disease, use the chart below to determine which grid most applies to your biopsy report. If you fall into the favorable parameters group, low Gleason's score and low volume of disease, and you want to purse a less aggressive treatment, it is reasonable to do so. However, if you are in the unfavorable parameters group, you may need to put aside your concerns about the ease of treatment or impact on your daily life in favor of choosing the more aggressive therapy with the most options for cure. (You can do radiation after surgery, but it is difficult to do surgery after radiation.)You need to know the parameters of your biopsy and the significance of each to help you in your decision. As you progress in your journey, you will begin to consider all the parameters, in addition to the specifics of your biopsy; which parameters you ultimately weigh most heavily in your decision can be determined only by you.

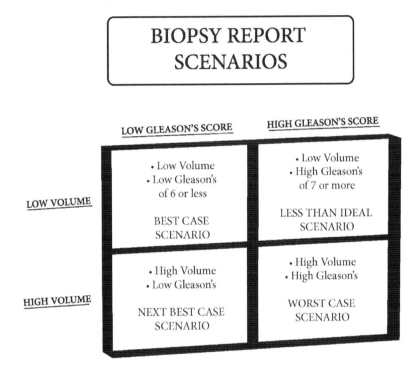

BIOPSY REPORT
SCENARIOS

	LOW GLEASON'S SCORE	HIGH GLEASON'S SCORE
LOW VOLUME	• Low Volume • Low Gleason's of 6 or less BEST CASE SCENARIO	• Low Volume • High Gleason's of 7 or more LESS THAN IDEAL SCENARIO
HIGH VOLUME	• High Volume • Low Gleason's NEXT BEST CASE SCENARIO	• High Volume • High Gleason's WORST CASE SCENARIO

The anatomy of the prostate - *Water and nerves*

Common things occur commonly.

Dramatic and life-threatening complications can occur with any of the forms of treatment for prostate cancer. Although knowledge of all potential problems and their likelihood should be part of your database in making "the decision," I recommend becoming familiar with the most common risks and side effects of the various treatments and weighing them more heavily in your decision-making process. *When you hear hoof beats, think horses, not zebras.* If you take all the uncommon, major risks off the table, you are left primarily with the effect the treatment you choose will have on how you void and your sexual function. This particular chapter is a primer on the prostate's anatomy and how it plays a role in the potential adverse effects of your treatment.

Water - *How the anatomy of the prostate relates to voiding.*

The prostatic urethra is the star of any prostate movie. Thee must know and understand the prostatic urethra regardless of the treatment chosen.

> All roads lead to Rome- All water flows through the prostatic urethra and the nerves loom nearby.

All treatments for prostate cancer affect the prostatic urethra. Surgical removal of the prostate removes the prostatic urethra and potentially causes activity related urinary incontinence. Radiation inflames the prostatic urethra and causes irritative urinary symptoms of frequency, urgency, getting up at night, and sometimes urgency incontinence. Choose your poison.

> Do you know where your prostatic urethra is tonight?

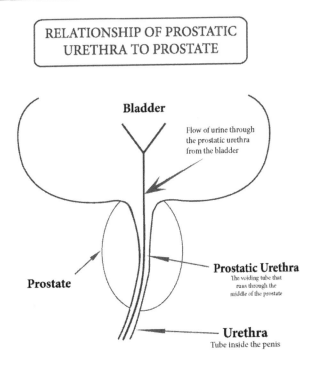

RELATIONSHIP OF PROSTATIC
URETHRA TO PROSTATE

Bladder

Flow of urine through
the prostatic urethra
from the bladder

Prostate

Prostatic Urethra
The voiding tube that
runs through the
middle of the prostate

Urethra
Tube inside the penis

When men urinate, the bladder contracts to force urine through the prostate and then out the urethra through the penis. Urine travels through a channel in the prostate called the prostatic urethra. As men age, usually starting around the age of 50, the prostate enlarges due to the male hormone testosterone. As the prostate enlarges, this "pinching in" from the lobes of the prostate narrows the prostatic urethra, making it more difficult to urinate. This difficulty voiding is common in older men, is more commonly associated with benign enlargement rather than cancer, and occurs earlier in some men than others.

The degree to which the prostate affects urinary flow varies as well. Almost all men will have some slowing of their urinary stream at some point in their life, but not all will feel that the severity of a less forceful stream requires treatment. In some men, the slowing progresses to the point that they cannot void at all (urinary retention). There are medicines for this that will either relax the muscles within the prostate to allow for better flow of urine or shrink the prostate to improve urinary flow. All of the treatment options for prostate cancer will affect how you void. It is incumbent upon you to know and anticipate the effects that various treatments will potentially have on how you void.

- *If the prostate is removed, then the prostatic urethra is removed. If your prostate is causing obstructive voiding symptoms, then the removal by surgery improves these symptoms.*

- *The voiding issues after surgery relate to the potential for incontinence as a result of the absence of the prostate and prostatic urethra.*

- *If you have radiation and already have obstructive voiding symptoms, these symptoms most probably will worsen.*

- *The voiding issues after radiation are caused by the inflammatory response of the prostatic urethra to the radiation. This results in the subsequent irritative or obstructive symptoms that commonly occur.*

Nerves - *You may have heard the expression, "I got one nerve, and you get on it!"*

> *You've got one nerve on each side of the prostate and all the treatments "get on em."*

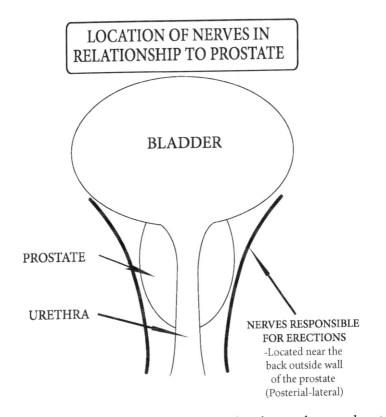

LOCATION OF NERVES IN
RELATIONSHIP TO PROSTATE

BLADDER

PROSTATE

URETHRA

NERVES RESPONSIBLE
FOR ERECTIONS
-Located near the
back outside wall
of the prostate
(Posterial-lateral)

The nerves responsible for erections in the male are located alongside the posterior-lateral aspect of the prostate. Surgical removal and radiation can both have a negative effect on these nerves, and hence both treatments can influence the subsequent quality of erections. With surgery, the nerves can be bruised or damaged in removing the prostate, and in the case of radiation, the nerves are damaged by the harmful effect of the radiation itself. Although both forms of therapy can affect the quality of the erection, the forms of treatment affect these nerves differently and in different time frames. For many men, the potential for a change in their ability to have an erection is the most important factor in choosing a treatment. It is very important for each man to first determine how much of a factor preserving erectile quality is for him. The patient then needs to understand specifically how the nerves will be affected by each treatment, keeping in mind his baseline function. The better a man's health and erectile function is before treatment, the better odds he has of preserving it regardless of the treatment chosen. In the risk-driven section of this book, the relationship between each treatment and its effect on these nerves will be presented in such a fashion as to help you place the "erection issue" in its proper place in the decision-making equation.

- *Surgery and radiation both affect the quality of the erection, but do so in different ways and in a different time frame.*

- *Choosing either treatment modality because you feel one is more certain to preserve your erections is a decision made in error.*

- *It is common to have the complete return to your baseline sexual function with surgery if the nerves are spared.*

- *You have a greater chance of complete loss of sexual function with surgery because of the irreparable harm done if both nerves are severed during surgery.*

- *Radiation will negatively affect your erection but to an unknown degree. You will not have a dramatic loss of your erectile quality, but a deleterious effect of the radiation on the nerves may occur over time.*

Treatment options - *A major inconvenience*

> # If a disease has several treatment options, then there is not one "good" one.

To highlight how difficult it is for many patients to decide what to do about their prostate cancer, consider the gallbladder. If it needs to be treated, there is one option: remove it. Once you decide to remove it, there is for the most part only one way it is removed: an hour-long laparoscopic outpatient procedure. If you have been having issues related to the digestive tract because of a sick gallbladder, all of those pesky symptoms go away once it is removed. Most patients are back to normal within a week or so.

Prostate cancer is very different. Prostate cancer has several treatment options and almost all will result in some change in voiding and/or sexual function. In addition to the concerns of the patient about whether he'll be cured or not, he has to worry about symptoms that are going to be caused by the treatment and not by the disease. The symptoms that can occur strike right at the heart of the male patient's pride (if he has debilitating voiding symptoms) and his sexuality (if his erections worsen). To make matters worse, some patients have favorable parameters indicating the slow-growing type of prostate cancer and may be completely symptom-free, but they are still faced with a decision about whether to undergo treatment. This patient is the one most troubled by the decision because he has to walk the fine line of limiting risks versus getting cured. He doesn't want to over-treat the cancer, subjecting himself to all the risks, but he doesn't want it to

come back either. Having prostate cancer, even low grade and low volume, is a lot like being a "little bit pregnant." Once you know you've got it, you have to deal with it (even if dealing with it is to choose surveillance). It is understandable why so many newly-diagnosed prostate cancer patients are frustrated by having to make the decision to pursue one treatment over another.

Though making a decision about which treatment to pursue is stressful, the vast majority of patients do well in terms of their prostate cancer and the treatment chosen. I often tell patients that they should expect the diagnosis and treatment to be a "major inconvenience" and the likelihood is that they will do fine and probably die of something other than prostate cancer. The trick is matching the patient to the right treatment and not allowing misconceptions or half-truths to drive the decision.

In order to come to a decision as to what form of treatment, if any, you want to pursue for your cancer, you need to understand the particulars of the various treatment options and how each will impact you. In addition, all the factors should be considered specifically as they apply to you. In medicine, decisions regarding a disease that has several available treatment options are the hardest to make. The decision regarding the treatment of your prostate cancer is no exception. I have spent hours with some patients over several weeks as they anguished over the pros and cons of the various treatment options in trying to decide which one was the best fit for them. To streamline the process, I am simplifying the treatment options to surgical removal of the prostate and radiation. Although some patients will choose cryosurgery (freezing the prostate), most patients choose between the various forms of radiation or surgery. Even if you are considering something other than these two major forms of treatment, the first decision is still whether you want to opt for surgical removal or something else. Your first task is to consider the big concept of "are you a surgery type or a radiation type?" Once this big decision is made, then the nuances of each particular treatment and its effects on you can be further considered. I will help you understand how characteristics about who you are and what is important to you are necessary ingredients in making "the decision." In addition, (by clarifying the potential risks of each treatment.) I will help you match the treatment to your particular situation and make your decision for the right reasons. Patients often latch on to one aspect of a treatment and make an ill-informed decision based on that alone, and my goal is to help you avoid that. Your decision should be based on numerous factors that are relevant only to you, meshed with the pros and cons of each of the options.

For the purposes of the following discussion, removal of the prostate, radioactive seed therapy (brachytherapy), and cryosurgery are operative procedures requiring anesthesia. Removal of the prostate (either by open surgery or by the robotic method) is more invasive, requires an incision or incisions, and has the highest associated operative risk. Unlike these treatments,, external beam radiotherapy is not considered an operative procedure, is similar to having 42 consecutive x-rays, and hence, for the most part, is not limited by the patient's underlying health.

All available treatments have the potential for risks. All of the treatments will affect how you void and the quality of your erection. In deciding on one form of treatment, the patient should have a clear understanding of the potential risks and which of those risks are most important to him. This allows the patient to match his decision to his particular health situation.

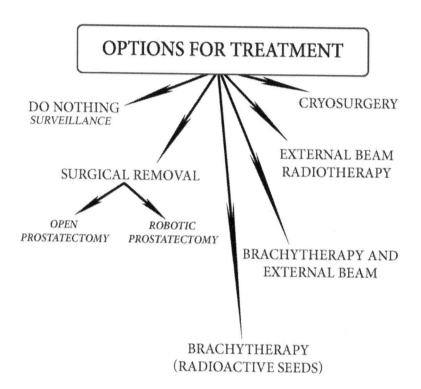

OPTIONS FOR TREATMENT

DO NOTHING
SURVEILLANCE

CRYOSURGERY

EXTERNAL BEAM
RADIOTHERAPY

SURGICAL REMOVAL

*OPEN
PROSTATECTOMY*

*ROBOTIC
PROSTATECTOMY*

BRACHYTHERAPY AND
EXTERNAL BEAM

BRACHYTHERAPY
(RADIOACTIVE SEEDS)

Life-threatening complications can occur in surgery, including blood loss, problems with anesthesia, postoperative infection, deep vein thrombosis, and heart attack, but these occur very rarely. Dramatic complications can also occur with radiation. Adverse effects on surrounding organs, problems with anesthesia (if you choose seeds), and other prolonged deleterious effects of the radiation can occur, but these also are uncommon. I have elected to discuss the problems that occur most commonly and those that patients deal with most frequently. The most common risks of surgery are the potential for incontinence or worsening of erectile function, and the most common risks of radiation are an exacerbation of obstructive voiding symptoms, initiation of irritative voiding symptoms, worsening of erectile function, and short and long-term problems related to the effect of radiation on the organs that surround the prostate (primarily the bladder and the bowel).

> # The worst thing that can happen to favorable short-term results is long-term follow up.

A patient of mine had recently been told his biopsy was positive for cancer, and he was in the office for the follow-up of his metastatic work-up (a C.T. scan looking for any lymph node involvement and a bone scan looking for bone involvement). In the middle of our discussion, I was called to the phone. When I returned a few moments later, the patient, a professor at a nearby college, had outlined all of the pros and cons of surgery and radiation on the exam table paper. It was very extensive and considered everything in terms of risks and options, with underlined words and arrows all over the paper. He was looking at what he had produced with his hand to his head as if he were pondering all the scenarios. I commended him for becoming so knowledgeable about prostate cancer and its treatments, but he said, "I am no closer to a decision than I was two weeks ago. This is tough." We talked some more, and he indicated he needed more time to decide. As we were leaving the room, he tore off the exam table paper, folded it nicely into a small square, and tucked it into his back pocket. I have him to thank for this particular chapter. He made me see how difficult it can be to arrive at a decision and, hence, the need for this book. He ultimately chose radiation therapy and had seeds without external beam radiation, and he did well. I saw this patient several months after his radiation to check his PSA and told him I was going to put the "exam table paper" anecdote in my book. He said, "I remember that; I still have that piece of paper." He then said something that surprised me: "Do you think I made the right decision?" Let me say it again, this decision is difficult, and there can be a lot of second-guessing even after the most thorough and thought-out decision. I told this patient that I did think he had made the right decision. He was certainly doing well in the short term. He had experienced only limited voiding symptoms and had dodged the early problems related to radiation, and that was a good start. Whether the cancer will come back and what effect the radiation will have on his sexual function are questions that will only be answered with time. This is another reason not to place too much emphasis on what someone else might recommend if he is in the short-term time frame of having had his own treatment. With prostate cancer, one must consider getting through the treatment itself and then weathering the aftermath of the treatment. One must know both the short-term and long-term consequences of all treatments to adequately make the decision; to consider one and not the other can lead to unhappy results.

When asked by a student a very intricate question regarding what treatment course should be advised to a newly diagnosed prostate cancer patient, the attending physician responded, "I don't believe I understand all I know about this disease."

"I don't believe I understand all I know about this disease."

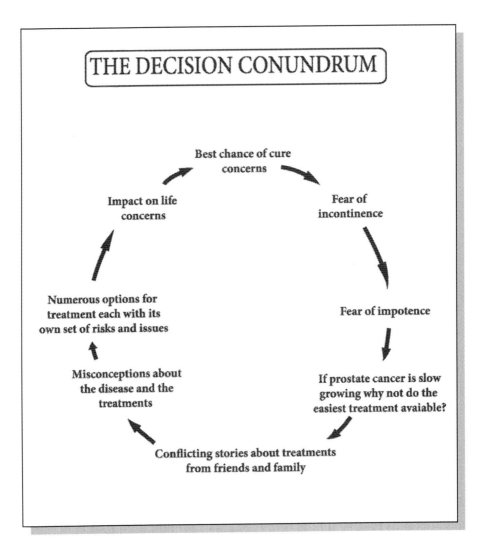

Part Two – "Who are you?" and why it matters

> *"Dr. McHugh, what would you advise me to do if I were your father?"*

I am asked this question very often after telling a family that a biopsy shows prostate cancer. I almost anticipate it and have to be careful not to smile after hearing it; certainly a smile after delivering bad news would come across as inappropriate. The irony of the question is that I am not a big fan of my father. He left my mother and her five boys when I was in the seventh grade and moved to Alaska. (That he went to Alaska reminds me of Jonah rejecting God's command to go to Nineveh. Jonah instead went to Tarshish; a location that was not only in the opposite direction but a "far and distant land." I have often thought that Alaska was my father's Tarshish.) I saw him only one time after that, when he showed up at my part-time job during the Christmas break of my freshman year in college. He quizzed me briefly about my grades, told me that his had been better at Auburn University, and then left. I never saw him again. After the divorce, my mother, brothers, and I moved to LaGrange, Georgia to live with my grandmother Bess Davis who was 73 at the time. Looking back on it, this was one of the best things that could have happened to me. LaGrange was a great place to grow up, I adored my mother and grandmother, and I feel that not having a father to depend on made me a stronger person. So, when the inevitable question comes up, I fight back the smile and answer the question as if it were a good one, in the context of a normal father-son relationship. Rarely, however, after failing to withhold the smile,

I've said, "That really is not the best question to ask me in light of my past relationship with my father. Considering the part of the male anatomy urologists work on, you might not like what I would recommend."

The decision of what treatment to choose is driven by several factors. It should be a decision that is tailored to you: "customized care," as I like to call it. A common question to the urologist is, "What would you do if you were me?" A better question would be, "Who am I, what is important to me, and what is best for me?" The answers to these questions will vary from person to person and, in turn, will influence their decisions. These personal differences often explain why two seemingly similar patients will choose widely different courses of treatment.

What follows is a breakdown of the important issues that will influence your decision; your job is to examine each in the context of your particular situation. This self-evaluation will aid you in understanding the factors that will ultimately drive your decision. To do this, it is important to know the factors that distinguish you as a patient (your "who are you" factors), your underlying voiding pattern and potency level, and how each treatment will affect each. As a urologist, I commonly see the voiding side effects of the treatments, and for that reason, a particular emphasis on this aspect of the decision is discussed. Every patient with prostate cancer who receives therapy will have some voiding side effects. Because all of the treatments will affect how you void differently, an emphasis the on mechanics of male voiding and how it is impacted by the various treatments is discussed in detail. It is imperative that you understand the different issues regarding how you void. This is delineated in the risk-driven section.

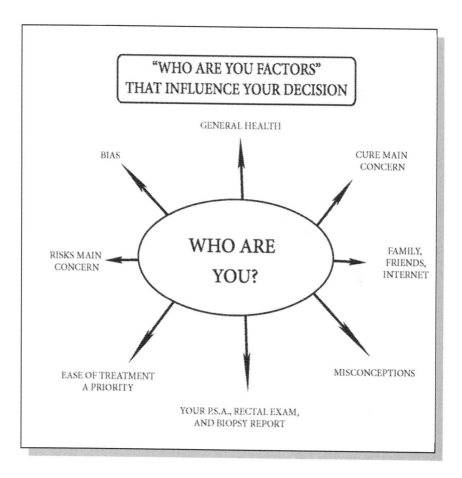

"WHO ARE YOU FACTORS" THAT INFLUENCE YOUR DECISION

GENERAL HEALTH

BIAS

CURE MAIN CONCERN

WHO ARE YOU?

RISKS MAIN CONCERN

FAMILY, FRIENDS, INTERNET

EASE OF TREATMENT A PRIORITY

MISCONCEPTIONS

YOUR P.S.A., RECTAL EXAM, AND BIOPSY REPORT

"Who are you?" factors

Each of these categories should be evaluated in the context of your particular situation and then used together to make your decision. The relative importance each will play in your decision-making process will be determined by you and will be unique to you. With time, you will combine these "who are you" factors with all of the information about your cancer and your assessment of risk versus cure to arrive at the decision that is best for *you.*

- General health, age, and years at risk

- Your PSA, rectal exam, and biopsy report

- Bias

- Cure is a priority

- Risks are a priority

- Ease of treatment is a priority

- What have you learned from family, friends, or the internet?

- Misconceptions about prostate cancer

General health, age, and years at risk - *What's best for the cancer may not be best for you.*

> ## If you live only by rules of thumb, you'll be all thumbs.

If you are in good health, all treatment options are available to you; however, if you have significant underlying health issues, your treatment options are more limited. A poor health scenario lends itself to the patient choosing either surveillance or external beam radiation.

An important concept regarding prostate cancer is that we think of survival rates in terms of 15 years. Other cancers, such as those that involve the breast or colon, are viewed in terms of 5-year survival rates. This difference is based on prostate cancer being, as a rule, a slow-growing cancer. I said "as a rule" because not all forms of prostate cancer are slow growing, which is why the specifics of the biopsy are important. The general perception that prostate cancer is slow-growing is sometimes used as an argument by patients who do not want to pursue a biopsy in the first place. The irony of this belief is that you have to have a biopsy to make the diagnosis of prostate cancer, and you need the results of the path report to know whether you have an aggressive (i.e. high Gleason's score) prostate cancer instead of the more common, slow-growing type. This mistaken belief, as well as the "I have no symptoms" argument, is often responsible for the delay in the diagnosis.

The effect of the 15-year survival concept of prostate cancer on your decision depends on your age and years at risk for recurrence of the disease. Using the years at risk concept in helping you make your decision usually results in the younger patient going for a more aggressive treatment and the older patient being less aggressive. Consider two patients with favorable biopsy results, one 75 years old and in marginal health, and the other 60 years old and in excellent health. If the biopsy indicates for both an 85% survival rate after 15 years, the older patient will likely either do nothing (surveillance) or choose the least invasive, least risky treatment option. In contrast, the 60-year-old patient will most likely be alive at 75. His years at risk are greater and risk of surgical complications is lower, thus he would be inclined toward more aggressive treatments. If cancer reoccurs after radiation, it usually does so within 5-8 years. Knowing this, a 75-year-old patient, if he elects to be treated at all, would pursue radiation under the assumption that if the cancer did return, he'd be well into his eighties and at risk for many other age-related medical problems. This is why patients will often offer up the commonly referenced half-truth, "Don't patients die *with* prostate cancer instead *of* dying of it?" In this case, the saying is correct for the 75-year-old, but it would not apply to a patient with more years at risk and/or more unfavorable parameters in his biopsy.

Physicians often evaluate the "physiologic" age rather than the chronological age of the patient. A 75-year-old man in good health, with no other medical problems and a family history of longevity, may have the physiologic age of a 65-year-old man. This age is also a factor that should be considered by the patient and doctor in making the decision.

- *How old are you and how does that impact your decision?*

- *How do your "years at risk" factor into your decision?*

- *What is your general health status? Do your operative risks for anesthesia and surgery outweigh the associated benefits?*

- *What insight might your family doctor provide about your operative risk?*

- *Which treatment options require anesthesia?*

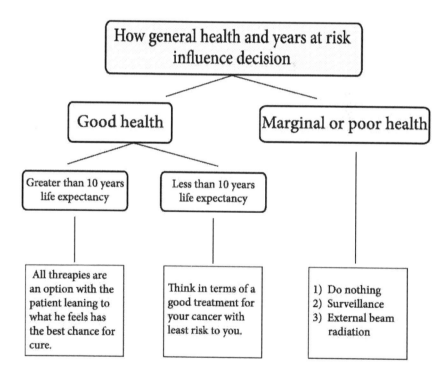

<u>*Your*</u> PSA, rectal exam and biopsy report – *Understanding the specifics of your disease is key to making the right decision.*

I had been checking my PSA for years and had watched it slowly creep up to just above normal. I decided to obtain a Free and Total PSA to see if it would offer any guidance regarding pursuing a biopsy. (In your blood, a portion of PSA is free (unbound), and a portion is bound by blood components. A low Free PSA indicates a higher possibility of a positive biopsy.) The day after my blood was drawn, my nurse Tina approached me with the lab report indicating a very low Free PSA.

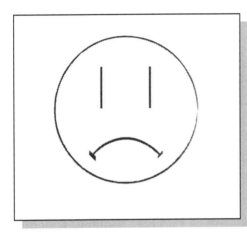

She had drawn a frowny face next to the lab value. I was crestfallen. "Tina, did you really have to put the little unsmiley face on it?" I decided at that moment that the time had come for me to have a prostate biopsy. I asked my partner to do it at lunch that very day, and the pathologist had the tissue samples in his hands by 1:30 p.m.

That evening my wife and I met at a little cabin we have on Lake Sidney Lanier, which is not uncommon on my half-day off on Thursdays. I had not told her that there was an issue with my PSA or that I had had a biopsy that day at lunch. I debated mentioning anything to her before I knew the biopsy results, but I chose to have her involved in the drama of waiting for the results and all the possibilities that entailed. "Karen, I had Bill do a biopsy on my prostate today. My PSA is slightly elevated, and I want to be sure that it doesn't mean I have a problem." (Remember, you don't start with the C word. You tell a patient and his wife, "There may be a problem with," " They found something," or "They have some concerns about...") We were sitting on the cabin's porch at the lake, and I had a panoramic view of the little piece of property where I spend a good portion of my weekends cutting grass, fishing, and working on the little vegetable garden we have there. My weekend ritual has become for our dog Chloe and me to pack up the trash in the back of my 1985 Toyota truck (my first car with air conditioning), take it to the county compactor, and then go to the lake. For years I have spent my weekends out there, always making a point to be home, as my mother would say, "by the time the street lights come on." As we were sitting there, out of nowhere, I said, "I don't really love this place Karen. I enjoy coming out here, but I don't really love it. I mean I wouldn't really miss it." She looked at me with disbelief. "What are you talking about John? You know you and Chloe love this place; are you thinking you are going to die or something? That's crazy." My wife (like most patients who have their prostates biopsied) didn't understand the possibility of having the "bad" kind of prostate cancer, the Frank Zappa kind. Frank Zappa died shortly after being diagnosed with inoperable prostate cancer, at the height of his musical career, in his 50s. That was my fear, and I will tell you it was real. As I pondered the possibilities of my pathology results, I gravitated to an acceptance that having the "slow-growing kind" of prostate cancer would be okay, but I prayed, "Please don't let me have the bad kind." If you have favorable parameters, you may die of prostate cancer, but it will take many years. If the biopsy has unfavorable parameters, the prognosis is unpredictable, with a higher likelihood of the cancer progressing quickly. I had seen this played out in patients of mine; I knew this, but my wife and family did not. I elected not to elucidate my concerns about the dual nature of prostate cancer to my wife; I had awakened her enough. This time period of "waiting on the results" really gets you thinking, and I was becoming very philosophical about my mortality, with a mentality of "what will be, will be" starting to set in.

I have included the PSA, rectal exam, and biopsy report in this section because now that you know the relative importance of each from the "basics" section, you now need to know the specifics of each as it pertains to you. These three issues play a major role in the "who are you" evaluation. Each of these has a favorable and unfavorable aspect that can influence your decision. The more favorable your parameters, the more options you have regarding treatment. A patient in his mid-70s with all favorable parameters might rightfully choose surveillance therapy. A younger patient may opt for a more aggressive treatment because of his years at risk. With all favorable parameters, he may elect to have external beam therapy. (This patient might have mild voiding symptoms, doesn't mind the 42 trips to the radiation center, and would prefer not to have surgery of any kind.) The favorable parameters give him options that might not be reasonable if all the parameters were of the more aggressive type. Your job is to find out each of these parameters by asking your physician the specifics of your case and then to use this information, along with other factors, to help in making your decision. When you leave the urologist's office with a diagnosis of prostate cancer, you should know your PSA, the specific findings of your rectal exam, and the grade (Gleason's score) and volume of disease (what percentage of the cores had cancer in them) on your biopsy report. You should also know the *significance* of each in order to appropriately make your decision. If you don't know or weren't told these aspects of your disease, ask. The diagram below shows how the results of the PSA, rectal exam, and biopsy report can be categorized as favorable or unfavorable:

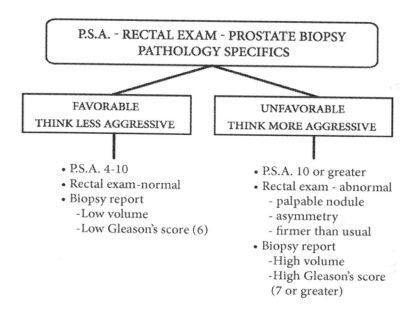

Bias – *Do you have a dog in this fight?*

> # If all you have is a hammer, the whole world is a nail.

*If the door of an elevator is closing, an internal medicine doctor will keep it from closing by placing his **hands** between the doors... A surgeon in the same situation will place his **head** between the doors.*

I have a friend, a surgeon, who, when I informed him that he had prostate cancer, immediately indicated to me that he wanted his prostate removed. He never questioned his decision from day one. His issue then became how to remove the prostate. As a surgeon he felt more comfortable following the surgeons' mantras: "Surgery separates the disease from the patient" and "A chance to cut is a chance to cure." Looking back, his quick decision exemplifies another saying about surgeons: "Sometimes wrong but never in doubt." When the father of another friend of mine, a radiation therapist, was diagnosed with prostate cancer, his son recommended radioactive seeds for his treatment and sent him to the institution where he had trained. This friend was more comfortable with radiation and more comfortable having the radiation administered by people he trusted at an institution with which he was familiar. Was one of these decisions more right or wrong than the other? No, but they do represent the prominent role that bias can play in deciding on a treatment for prostate cancer.

Often, upon learning that his path report shows prostate cancer, a patient will say quickly, "I want it out." Alternatively, his wife may immediately say, "I'd take it out, dear." This is an example of what I mean by bias: a preconceived gut feeling that directs your decision. Other patients have an "anti-surgery" bias and gravitate to non-surgical treatments from day one. If you have a bias, then other issues will not be as important to you in the decision-making process. *The patients who have an immediate bias in favor of a specific treatment have the least tormented time reaching their decision, but this does not mean they make a better one.*

Physicians can also be biased. Be wary if your physician pushes too strongly for his or her particular specialty in making recommendations. (As a surgeon myself, I feel that I am also biased to a degree, but only in the context of certain parameters. The ultimate decision is yours.)

Keep in mind the saying, "If all you have is a hammer, the whole world is a nail." In other words, the surgeon recommends surgery, the radiation therapist recommends radiation, and the used car salesman recommends his used cars. All the options regarding the various treatment modalities should be given to you in an unbiased fashion. You can then apply what you've learned about those modalities to what is important to you and what you feel is best for your particular situation. With all this in hand, you can make an informed decision without letting your bias, or that of your physician, play a more prominent role than is prudent.

- *Do you have a bias toward which treatment you feel is best for you?*

- *Do you have a fear of surgery?*

- *Does the idea of an incision or wearing a urethral catheter bother you?*

- *Does the idea of radiation in your body scare you?*

- *Do you feel your urologist is biased toward surgery?*

- *Do you feel the radiation therapist is biased toward radiation?*

Cure–driven – *Most aggressive treatment is your priority*

Patients who choose surgery usually think of cure as the most prominent issue and have adopted an attitude of "damn the torpedoes" regarding concerns about risk and inconvenience.

Patients often choose radiation not because they think it is the best treatment for curing their cancer, but because it is the treatment that best balances cure with risk and inconvenience. In essence, they are betting on radiation to allow them to "have their cake and eat it too."

Prostate cancer
in many respects
is very different
from other
cancers; patients
will often value
ease of treatment
over a primary
concern for
curative results.

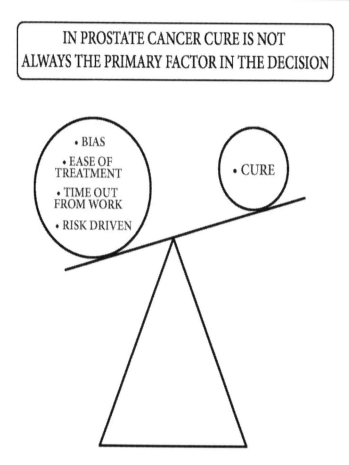

IN PROSTATE CANCER CURE IS NOT ALWAYS THE PRIMARY FACTOR IN THE DECISION

- BIAS
- EASE OF TREATMENT
- TIME OUT FROM WORK
- RISK DRIVEN

- CURE

I initially wanted to have my prostate cancer treated by seed therapy. (This is how serious I was in considering this form of therapy): I was evaluated by a radiotherapist, catheterized, and had prostate ultrasound for mapping one day during lunch. To be more graphic, that's an ultrasound probe in the rectum and a catheter in the penis, quite the lunchtime experience. Seeds appealed to me because of my concerns regarding time off from work. I would have been able to have the seeds placed on a Friday and then return to work on Monday. For most doctors and other patients diagnosed during their working years, not being at work is a triple whammy: you are not making any income, the overhead

marches on, and you are spending money while you are off.
Despite these concerns, being cured became my most pressing
issue over time. As I inquired more about seeds, I was advised that
the quality of the placement of the seeds was paramount to getting
an adequate treatment and hence cure. There was room for error.
It concerned me that if I did not have a procedure with good
placement, then my cancer was likely to return due to my young
age at diagnosis and my years at risk. In surgery, unless the cancer
extends to the edge of the prostate, complete removal is not as
operator-dependent as is the appropriate placement and
distribution of the radioactive seeds. Sparing of the nerves is
operator-dependent, while removing the whole gland at the time of
prostatectomy is generally not a concern. As I got closer to my
decision, concern over the variable of seed placement and how it
related to cure was an important factor to me and moved my
decision toward surgical removal.

It may seem obvious that a patient would always choose the
treatment which he feels has the highest chance of curing his
cancer. In prostate cancer, however, the cure rates of the two most
common modalities, removing the prostate (radical prostatectomy)
and radiation therapy (external beam, seeds, or a combination of
both) have very similar survival rates after 15 years. Because the
cure rates are similar, patients begin to investigate which of the
treatment options will impact their life the least. It is not
uncommon for a patient to get bogged down in the balancing act of
weighing cure rates against the potential for complications and
changes in his quality of life. Let's say that you are of the opinion
that removing the prostate will give you the very best shot at being
cured and you are of the age and health to safely undergo the
procedure. You soon learn that surgical removal is complicated by

the need for anesthesia, hospitalization, an incision, a catheter, postoperative incontinence requiring protection, and time out from work. That is the dilemma of surgery; you may feel it gives you the best chance of cure, but there are more initial hurdles and hoops to jump through. When a patient begins to examine the options and learns of the potential for the complications associated with surgical removal, ease of treatment will often become the most important factor in "the decision." It is this issue that is highlighted in mass mailed radioactive seed brochures showing a man as a patient one week and playing golf with friends, smiling, the next.

Surgical removal differs from radiation in that it allows for the pathological evaluation of the removed prostate to determine definitively the volume of cancer, if there is extension of the cancer beyond the prostate's outer capsule, and Gleason's grade. The final surgical pathology can be different from what you might have expected from the biopsy report; it is not uncommon for the surgical pathology report to show a more extensive cancer than the biopsy results implied. This is referred to as upstaging. The final pathology report gives the patient and surgeon more information regarding prognosis and the true extent of the disease in the prostate, but is not necessarily a reason to choose surgery. The true extent and grade of the prostate cancer will not be known if radiation is chosen; if the prostate is not removed, it cannot be pathologically evaluated.

If your cancer is confined to the gland only, there are fewer variables for failure of the treatment, as it pertains to curing you of your disease, with surgery than with radiation.

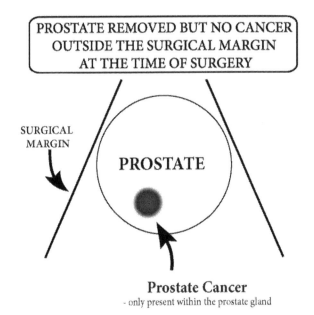

Prostate Cancer
- only present within the prostate gland

If a person has his prostate removed and the cancer was completely confined to the prostate, there is a high likelihood that his cancer is cured, although, as with any type of cancer, cures cannot be guaranteed. Incomplete removal of the prostate, leaving a small amount of prostate behind harboring cancer cells, occurs infrequently and is usually not an issue. I use "high likelihood," because some patients will mistakenly choose surgery thinking that there is sure cure with removal, but this is a misconception. Surgical removal of the prostate obviously will not address cancer cells that have migrated out of the prostate prior the procedure and hence can lead to disease recurrence. In the case of radiation, there is the same risk that cancer cells are present outside the prostate and treatment field; these cancer cells evade treatment as well. In addition, there is always the small chance that either the radiation dose isn't sufficient to kill all the cancer in the prostate or, in the case of brachytherapy, the seeds are placed in such a way as to leave a small, untreated portion of the prostate harboring cancer, a "skip area."

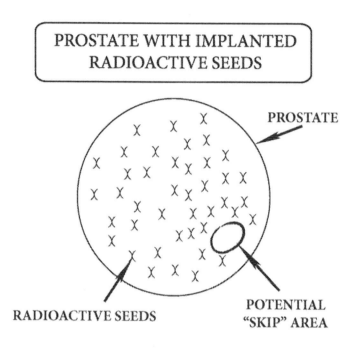

PROSTATE WITH IMPLANTED RADIOACTIVE SEEDS

PROSTATE

RADIOACTIVE SEEDS

POTENTIAL "SKIP" AREA

It is better to cure at the beginning than at the end; or... if you only had one shot at it what would you do?

Patients will often ask, "If the prostate has been removed, then how can the PSA go up?" The following diagram explains this phenomenon. If your PSA rises after surgery, local spread of cancer cells occurred prior to your treatment. If your PSA rises after radiation, there is an additional possibility that the radiation did not kill all the cancer inside the prostate. If you have the prostate removed and later your PSA begins to rise (i.e. a small amount of cancer was outside the gland before removal), you still can have the option of a full course of external beam radiation, offering you a second chance at cure with less volume of disease to treat. In addition to this, patients tolerate radiation better and have fewer voiding symptoms related to radiation after having had the prostate removed.

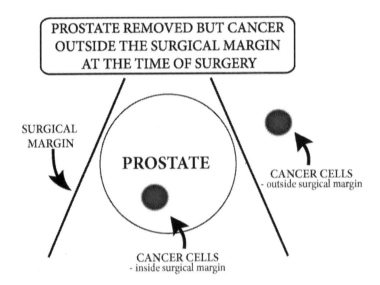

Whereas you can safely treat a patient who has had the surgical removal of the prostate at a later time with radiation; following radiation with surgical removal is more complicated. If your PSA rises after radiation, (i.e. the cancer was either outside the prostate before radiation or the radiation did not kill it),surgical removal of the prostate is possible, but it is performed in only a few centers in the country and with much higher complication rates because of the changes in the tissue planes that occur with radiation. In my 22 years practicing urology, I have not had a patient with recurrent prostate cancer who opted for surgical removal of the prostate after having received radiation. If you choose radiation treatment, your surgical options for dealing with any of the complications associated with radiation, particularly obstructive voiding symptoms, are also limited, which will be discussed in more detail later. These factors, more than the ability to cure, are the caveats of radiation therapy that I feel are most often overlooked by patients choosing seed therapy.

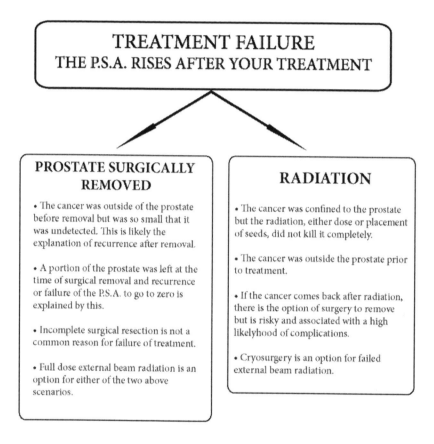

Patients who elect to have radiation usually do not do so because they think the cure rate is better; their feeling is that the cure will be just as good without all the hassle of surgery. Most patients who have the prostate removed think it will be the most aggressive way to treat the cancer. Neither rationale is necessarily flawed, but each patient should look at all the other factors and envision how they will be doing clinically down the road after the initial trials of the treatment, whether surgery or radiation, are over. The decision should not be one-dimensional. If a patient chooses radiation because it's easy and yet has significant underlying voiding issues, he probably made the wrong decision. If a patient who has heart disease is adamant about surgery, he should consider the risks related to the procedure and the possibility of peri-operative complications. This is what I mean in saying that what may be best for treating the cancer may not be best for the patient.

> • *Are cure and increased options for other forms of therapy in the face of a post-treatment rising PSA the driving forces in making your decision?*

> • *Does the ease of treatment (no catheter, no incision, and shorter recovery time) override your concerns regarding cure and the availability of future surgical options?*

> • *If the cancer is only in the gland and the gland is removed then you are cured. This is not always the case with radiation. Does this influence your decision?*

Risk-driven – *Least chance of side effects is your priority*

What may be best for the cancer may not be the best thing for you.

Pay me now or pay me later.
There is no free ride.

I was in the midst of the confusion over what to do and which treatment to pursue, when I saw a patient in my office, aged 63 and in good general health, whose PSA was now rising six years after having had brachytherapy. On the day of that office visit, he was on his way to a granddaughter's birthday party. I realized then, considering that I was 52, I did not want to be in the situation of having a rising PSA ten years later and feeling that I had not done "the most I could do" in treating my cancer. I decided that the increased likelihood of being cured with surgery was more important to me than the risks and complications associated with it. On that day, after months of deliberation, I decided that I would have my prostate removed. I felt very strongly that if I had any of the problems associated with surgery, so be it. "Damn the torpedoes! Full speed ahead!" ("Damn the torpedoes! Full speed ahead!" is attributed to U.S. Navy Admiral Farragut during the Civil War Battle of Mobile Bay.)

It is my feeling that surgery is a cleaner process, and I knew that once I got over the surgery, the catheter, and the frustration of post-operative incontinence, I would not have the

> I felt then as I do now, that surgical removal assures that all the cancer in the prostate will be gone; radiation of the prostate cannot assure you that all the cancer in the gland will be killed.

unknown of the potential side effects common to radiation. I preferred paying up front for the known complications of surgery to paying later for the unknown side effects of radiation. A secondary factor for me was the fact that I was already having mild to moderate obstructive voiding symptoms, and surgical removal would eliminate the potential for future problems with voiding. For me, concern regarding the possibility of total incontinence, which can happen after surgery, was outweighed by what I felt was a better chance of cure and the prevention of the almost certain worsening of my already symptomatic prostate enlargement.

Both *radiation and surgical removal* affect how you void and the quality of your erection.

All men treated for prostate cancer will experience a change in how they void. How he will void is rarely considered by the patient adequately. You can often predict the potential for voiding problems after treatment by accurately assessing the voiding pattern before treatment. If a patient makes a decision without careful consideration of his underlying voiding pattern and how it will potentially be affected, neither he nor the doctor has done his due diligence. A desire to highlight the importance of this issue when choosing a treatment option played a large role in my decision to write this book. I am, like other urologists, very familiar with the side effects of radiation on how men void, because it is often the urologist, not the radiation therapist, who manages post-radiation patients with voiding problems.

You urinate several times a day; you probably have sex much less frequently. Treatments affect both functions, so it makes sense to make decisions based on which side effect will impact the quality of your life the most. Not all men have good erections when they are diagnosed with prostate cancer, and, hence, salvaging sexual function may not be a primary factor in their decision. If potency is not a major factor in the decision process, then the importance of how the treatment chosen will affect voiding becomes much more important. After careful consideration, a younger patient may well value the potential for a change in his sexual function more than a change in how he voids. These issues need to be fully vetted and considered early on in the decision journey.

Good cooking is remembered long after the sex is gone.

> Could it be true for you that how well you pee is remembered long after the sex is gone?

How you void - Abnormal voiding patterns in males and why they are important to "the decision".

It is imperative that you understand the abnormal voiding patterns in males and the influence of the various treatments on each of them. A decision made by you regarding treatment without consideration of the following issues is a decision made in error. Both surgical removal and radiation, particularly in the form of radioactive seeds, will affect how you void. Incontinence can be an issue with both, but in different forms. To understand how radiation or surgery will affect how you will void, you must have a working knowledge of the abnormal voiding patterns that can result from treatment:

• Obstructive urinary symptoms
• Irritative urinary symptoms
• Incontinence

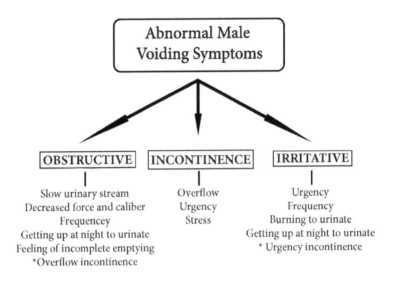

An enlarged prostate can manifest itself by causing either irritative or obstructive urinary symptoms. In some men, the first symptoms related to enlargement of the prostate are irritative, including nocturia (getting up at night), urgency to void, frequency, or dysuria (a burning that occurs with voiding). Irritative symptoms occur because the bladder is working harder to bypass the enlarging prostate's obstructive effect on the prostatic urethra. The effect of the enlarged prostate pushing up on the bladder makes the bladder more sensitive to certain foods and drinks that contain irritants such as caffeine or acid, and this contributes to irritative voiding symptoms. Other men have obstructive urinary symptoms (caused by the narrowing of the prostatic urethra), which are characterized by a slow stream or a urinary stream that is decreased in force and caliber. They may notice that it takes them longer to empty their bladder or have a sensation of incomplete emptying. Some men have both irritative and obstructive symptoms due to their enlarging prostate.

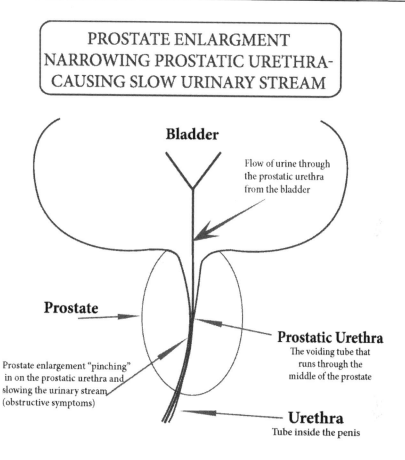

PROSTATE ENLARGMENT NARROWING PROSTATIC URETHRA-CAUSING SLOW URINARY STREAM

Bladder

Flow of urine through the prostatic urethra from the bladder

Prostate

Prostate enlargement "pinching" in on the prostatic urethra and slowing the urinary stream (obstructive symptoms)

Prostatic Urethra
The voiding tube that runs through the middle of the prostate

Urethra
Tube inside the penis

It is unusual for men to have incontinence (uncontrolled leakage of urine) unless their irritative symptoms cause urgency incontinence (the urge is so bad that one cannot get to a restroom in time) or overflow incontinence (the obstruction is so severe that the bladder can't empty; it overflows as a dribble into the prostatic urethra and then out the tip of the penis). A thorough understanding of how a man voids normally and with the various degrees of enlargement is important to the patient with prostate cancer considering his options because the baseline voiding pattern will be impacted differently depending on the treatment chosen.

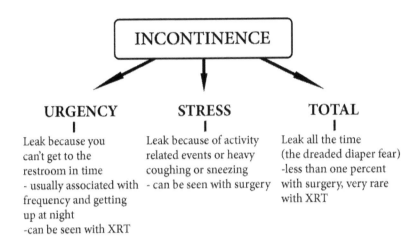

INCONTINENCE

URGENCY	STRESS	TOTAL
Leak because you can't get to the restroom in time - usually associated with frequency and getting up at night -can be seen with XRT	Leak because of activity related events or heavy coughing or sneezing - can be seen with surgery	Leak all the time (the dreaded diaper fear) -less than one percent with surgery, very rare with XRT

Because radiation inflames the prostatic urethra, it can initiate irritative and obstructive symptoms that were not present pretreatment and will probably worsen any underlying voiding symptoms already present. Surgery, because it removes the prostate and the prostatic urethra, will improve obstructive symptoms, but has the risk of causing total or stress urinary incontinence. Stress incontinence occurs with straining, coughing, sneezing, or any activity that increases abdominal pressure and, in turn, forces urine to leak out of the bladder. This is rare in a male unless he has had the prostate removed. After surgical removal of the prostate, the male depends on the muscles around the bladder (the external sphincter) to maintain continence. Total incontinence occurs if the external sphincter is damaged at the time of prostate removal (unusual) or if the patient's anatomy is such that the function of the external sphincter alone is not enough to ensure continence. Total incontinence occurs uncommonly after surgery and very rarely after radiation.

A man spends his first 50 years trying to make money, his second 50 trying to make water.

- *What is my baseline voiding pattern; is it normal, obstructive or irritative?*

- *Have I accurately assessed how I void and considered this in my decision?*

- *Does the ease of treatment associated with radiation, but with the possibility of irritative voiding symptoms or worsening of underlying obstructive symptoms that cannot be treated surgically, trump for you the benefits, the risks, and inconveniences of surgery?*

- *Can you differentiate the types of incontinence and voiding patterns and how each is affected by the various treatments?*

- *What would bother your more, occasional stress incontinence which can occur with surgery, or the irritative symptoms of frequency, urgency, and getting up more at night which can occur with radiation?*

Radiation

Around the tube (prostatic urethra) in your prostate, through which you urinate, will be placed 80 to 100 radioactive seeds, and in some cases external beam radiation will also be treating this area. Does it surprise you that there will be a "how you void" consequence to this?

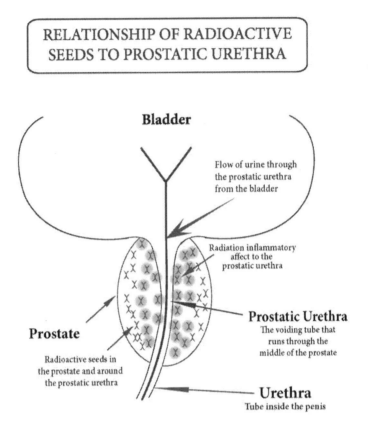

RELATIONSHIP OF RADIOACTIVE SEEDS TO PROSTATIC URETHRA

Bladder

Flow of urine through
the prostatic urethra
from the bladder

Radiation inflammatory
affect to the
prostatic urethra

Prostatic Urethra
The voiding tube that
runs through the
middle of the prostate

Prostate

Radioactive seeds in
the prostate and around
the prostatic urethra

Urethra
Tube inside the penis

Radiation causes irritative symptoms secondary to the radiation's effect on the bladder and, more importantly, its effect on the prostatic urethra. As previously discussed, the prostate has a channel through the middle of it that urine goes through after leaving the bladder called the prostatic urethra. Radiation irritates and inflames the tissue lining the prostatic urethra. This effect is more pronounced with seeds than with external beam radiation. The subsequent effect of radiation on the prostatic urethra gives one the sensation of needing to void and causes, in varying degrees, urgency, frequency, getting up at night to void more often, or a burning sensation when voiding. In severe cases, the urge to void is so intense and urgent that incontinence occurs because of the patient not being able to reach the bathroom in time (urgency incontinence). The severity of these irritative symptoms and how long they last vary from patient to patient. It is difficult to predict how it will affect each individual person. A patient won't know to what degree the irritative symptoms will affect him until he has actually had the radiation. *This is why one day a patient will tell me he wants radiation because a friend did so well, and the next another tells me adamantly that he does not want radiation because of all the side effects a friend had.* Some patients have significant symptoms for a long time, others minor symptoms for a short period of time. In the case of urinary symptoms related to radiation that don't resolve with medicines, a watch and wait therapy is usually recommended because most of these symptoms resolve or abate with time to varying degrees. As shown later in the representative case studies section, surgical intervention by a urologist is a last-resort option in this scenario because of the problems related to operating on irradiated tissues.

If a patient is having difficulty with the force or caliber of his urinary stream before radiation (obstructive symptoms), these symptoms will also probably worsen, (particularly with seeds). The inflammation that occurs as a result of the radiation aggravates the underlying problem of the prostatic tissue encroaching on the prostatic urethra. In fact, I am now very sensitive, as are most radiation oncologists, in delineating the patients with an underlying obstructive voiding pattern if radiation is the modality chosen. If you are on a medicine to help you void better, either the one that shrinks the prostate or the one that relaxes it, you might be at heightened risk for worsening of your obstructive symptoms following radiation. Something important to consider is that if you do have obstructive symptoms after radiation, most of the surgical options that the urologist would normally utilize to relieve the inability to void cannot be done without an attendant increased risk of making things worse.

Once you have chosen radiation, you have limited surgical options to correct any worsening of your ability to void. You are" attached at the hip" with it, both from the standpoint of surgical intervention of any urinary symptoms that occur as well as for curative measures if your PSA rises, indicating return of the cancer.

If you have had radiation and are unable to void at all, i.e. urinary retention, then you would need to wear a catheter or self-catheterize yourself until you could void. If you are the unfortunate patient who has to wear a catheter after radiation therapy, the usual advice is to wait it out and have voiding trials (take the catheter out and see if you can void; if you can't, replace it) until you can urinate again. This time frame varies from days to months and from patient to patient. Medicines can be utilized, but usually not surgery. The "tincture of time" is usually the treatment for symptoms secondary to radiation. If in your evaluation of your voiding pattern you determine you have red flags, particularly obstructive voiding symptoms, it is better to deal with them before radiation than after. You can open the prostatic urethra before radiation with transurethral microwave therapy or laser prostatectomy, but not after.

> Again... It is better to cure at the beginning than at the end.

Surgery

The biggest fear of patients regarding the surgical removal of the prostate gland is total incontinence, or leaking urine all the time. The "will I have to wear a diaper" question or fear of this complication drives the decision for many patients. Prior to the Walsh nerve sparing radical prostatectomy, total incontinence was relatively common; however, total incontinence today occurs in less than 1% of patients. It is more common to have stress incontinence, that which occurs with heavy activity, coughing or sneezing. In my opinion, the fear of total incontinence resulting from removal of the prostate should not be viewed as the major issue in the decision. However, if the possibility of stress incontinence, which occurs to varying degrees in patients who have the prostate removed, concerns you and is a decision driver, then surgery may not be for you.

Prior to surgical removal of the prostate the male's continence depends on the bladder neck, the prostatic urethra, and the external sphincter. As seen in the diagram that follows, after surgical removal of the prostate, the male depends primarily on the external sphincter. This dependence on the external sphincter and the heightened role it now plays are very similar to the anatomical situation found in the female. (Girls don't have a prostate.) This also explains why it is not uncommon to have varying degrees of stress incontinence, which occurs commonly in females, in some post-prostatectomy patients.

> **After the prostate is removed, the male anatomy from a urinary standpoint becomes much like that of a female. The male's continence now depends on the external sphincter.**

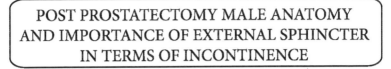

POST PROSTATECTOMY MALE ANATOMY
AND IMPORTANCE OF EXTERNAL SPHINCTER
IN TERMS OF INCONTINENCE

BLADDER-PROSTATE-URETHRA   BLADDER-URETHRA
Before Surgical Removal of Prostate   After Surgical Removal of Prostate

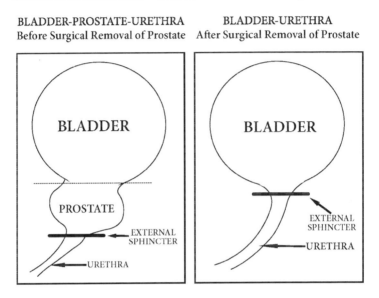

Contrary to the various radiation treatments, having obstructive urinary symptoms prior to surgery is not a negative, but a positive factor for choosing surgical removal. The removal of the prostate treats the cancer and at the same time corrects the obstructive nature of the prostate. In men with a new diagnosis of prostate cancer who have obstructive urinary symptoms, the obstructive symptoms are usually related to prostate enlargement and not to the cancer itself. Obstructive symptoms, when caused by prostate cancer, are usually indicative of a very aggressive, locally extensive prostate cancer. This is true because most prostate cancers are in the posterior aspect of the prostate (the portion that can be felt with a rectal exam), and this area is well away from the prostatic urethra, and hence they cause no voiding symptoms.

In my practice, and it may be true with all caregivers, nothing is more detrimental to the early detection of prostate cancer than the misconception that if a man has no voiding symptoms, he must not have cancer. In regards to prostate cancer education, correction of this errant perception is probably job number one.

THE REASON THERE ARE NO VOIDING SYMPTOMS WITH EARLY PROSTATE CANCER

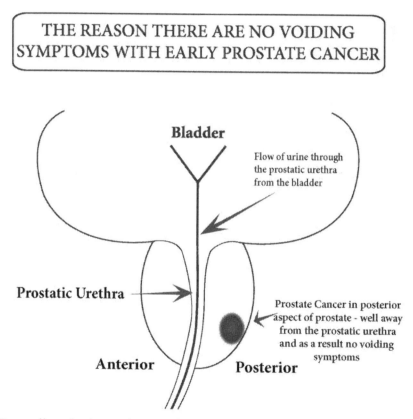

Bladder

Flow of urine through the prostatic urethra from the bladder

Prostatic Urethra

Prostate Cancer in posterior aspect of prostate - well away from the prostatic urethra and as a result no voiding symptoms

Anterior   Posterior

Regarding the incontinence that a patient experiences after surgery, the time to being continent after removal of the catheter varies. I have had patients who were dry from the very day the catheter was removed and others for whom it took several months. This will be clearly emphasized to you by your urologist, and as you begin your decision journey, you will probably weigh this possibility heavily. For reasons we don't understand, the time to continence varies from patient to patient, despite a properly performed prostatectomy. Total incontinence that persists is very uncommon, but stress incontinence occurs fairly commonly. You have to decide how important this is to you, and if a fear of this is great, then you may not choose surgery. Just as the radiation therapist cannot tell you how your body will respond to radiation, the surgeon cannot tell you the timing of when you will become continent, and if or to what degree you will have stress incontinence.

I was totally incontinent for about three months. I initially thought that diapers would manage the problem, but even the most absorbent brand would last only 45 minutes without getting heavy and beginning to sag down between my legs. I went back to work with a full patient load 11 days after my surgery. It quickly became apparent that a diaper alone would not work. Going back and forth to the restroom in between every four or five patients got old very quickly. I then tried the technique of adding an absorbent liner inside the diaper and only changing that, but the liner was cumbersome as well, and still I had to dispose of and replace it several times a morning. I soon found that the only thing that would let me have freedom from all the paraphernalia related to diapers was a condom catheter. We used to joke as urology residents, saying, "I'm going to go empty my leg bag," instead of saying we were going to go to the restroom. There were residents who would take condom catheters from the urology clinic and put them on at baseball games so they could drink beer without the inconvenience of going to the stadium restroom. I ordered several types to try out (I won't tell which size I ultimately used) and actually got along quite well with them. The ones I used were like a condom with sticky glue on the inner surface. As you roll it on, it sticks to the skin and forms a water-tight seal; the end of it has a spout that connects to a tube and a bag that attaches to a leg, hence the term "leg bag." I could wear this under my scrubs and no one knew I had it on. I worked in the office, operated, and even taught youth Sunday school with this set-up undetected. This system malfunctioned and popped open only once. This soaked the pant leg of the scrubs I was wearing, but no one saw it and I was able to correct that quickly with a new pair of scrub bottoms. There was an ever-present fear that it might leak at an inopportune time, but that never happened. I had told very few people that I had had my prostate removed, so hardly anyone knew that I had a "leakage" issue and was wearing a leg bag. I would be speaking to a patient about what they should do for their prostate and answering questions about incontinence, all the while wearing my leg bag. It was an odd time; I elected not to tell patients about my situation. I bet in those three months of wearing protection that I must have treated hundreds of patients with prostate issues. "What would you do if it were you?" they would ask as I could feel my leg bag filling up. The bag holds about a pint, so I could feel it getting heavy and bulging the scrubs at the calf level of my leg. If you let the bag get too full, then it begins to pull down on the tubing, which in turns pulls down on the condom, which pulls down on the... You get the picture. With time, as I am sure it is with most inconveniences that patients endure, all of the issues associated with the condom catheter became second nature, just part of my life.

I would take off the condom before my shower and then jump around to see if the leaking had improved, and each morning for those three months, I was disappointed. Following the shower, I would dry the area to perfection and then carefully roll on my condom catheter and begin the process of hooking everything up. I had a routine that took about 15 minutes. On one particular morning, some of the skin of my "you know what" was very irritated and little blisters were all over the skin, particularly where urine would contact inside the condom. The condom catheter's glue made taking off the condom a very unpleasant experience, as it would pull at the irritated areas of skin and open the blisters as well. It was very painful to take off the old and miserable to then put on the new. I remember being quite depressed by my situation that morning, more so than usual. As if it were not bad enough to be leaking all the time, now my system for dealing with it was also problematic. The thought of wearing this contraption all day, considering all the movement and discomfort that this entailed, also added to my despondency. The other issue was that if the skin kept getting irritated, I would not be able to use the condom catheter and would have to go back to diapers. I was pondering my plight and was just about "situated" when my wife entered our master bath. I was stooped over in order to connect the rubber straps of the bag to my calf and looked up at her. She looked at me oddly and with what I perceived as a look of concern. I thought that maybe she had detected my frustration and slight depression. I remember being disappointed that my true feelings might have been revealed, as I had been trying to down-play to my family the pathetic "urinary" situation that had become my life. By the way she peered down at me I was sure she was going to ask, "Is everything O.K?" She then said," John, I think I see a black hair on the tip of your nose." Somewhat relieved, as I connected the last leg strap, I said, "Thank you dear."

I remember I was working in the backyard, and for the first time in months I felt the urge to void. As urine had been just passing through my bladder, this was significant. Just like that, no warning, it just happened. "Karen guess what? I just urinated!" From that point on for about a week I could get by with a diaper a day. I came to love my diapers, they were comfortable, had perforated breathable sides, and just using one pair a day was not very different from wearing underwear. Not having to roll on the sticky condom catheter every morning was like being set free and being in heaven. I told my wife that, if I had to, being "dry with a diaper and potent with a pill" was a situation that I could live with forever. I made up a little jingle that I would sing with those words, as I'd do a jig in front of the bathroom mirror. I also had a "routine" where I'd say that I could be a poster boy for Depends and maybe be the model for a new line of diapers for active and professional men hiding the fact that they leaked but led a productive life. (I had in mind diapers with little fly-fishermen on them.) This shows you how a patient's frame of mind changes, and how what is important to you evolves throughout your journey with medical issues.

Comparing radiation to surgery in the context of incontinence

- Irritative symptoms are very common after radiation, very uncommon with surgery.

- That you have no urinary symptoms is for the most part irrelevant in prostate cancer detection or treatment. If you have symptoms they can serve as important factors in the treatment chosen.

• Total incontinence (leaking urine all the time) is something to consider if choosing to have surgical removal, but because it occurs uncommonly, it should not be the main factor in the decision.

• Total incontinence is very rare with radiation and occurs in less than one percent of patients with surgery.

• Obstructive voiding symptoms are worsened by radiation and improved by surgery.

• Stress incontinence can occur with surgery and is uncommon with radiation. Urgency incontinence as a result of pronounced irritative symptoms can occur with radiation and is uncommon with surgery.

• The irritative symptoms associated with radiation and the stress incontinence seen with surgical removal can improve with time.

• There are surgical options available for the uncommon occurrence of total incontinence seen with surgery; however, there are limited surgical options for the irritative or obstructive symptoms after radiation. There are medications that help with the symptoms caused by radiation.

• All of the urinary symptoms that are common with radiation are worse for seeds than for external beam. The combination of seeds and external beam radiation obviously has a greater negative effect on how you void than either of the two modalities alone.

• Radiation cystitis and other problems associated with radiation can develop several years after the treatment (a "pay me later" factor you should consider).

On the following page you will find a fairly comprehensive flow (no pun intended) chart of abnormal male voiding patterns. As a urologist I see these patterns daily, particularly in patients who have been treated for prostate cancer. As I have stated previously, it is imperative that you understand the characteristics of each symptom listed. Regardless of the treatment you choose, you **_will_** have one or more of the following voiding issues. How long they will last or how severe they will be for you is an unknown. Your job is to not only understand these urinary symptoms, but to be knowledgeable of which treatment is most often associated with and most likely to cause them. You then should evaluate your current voiding pattern, and in advance of any treatment or decision, determine which complex of urinary symptoms you will be likely to have. This exercise in turns aids you in your decision. An attempt to clarify and make known to the reader how these "how you void" issues are affected by the common treatments of prostate cancer was a major impetus for writing this book. Trust me…this is important.

.

There **_will be_** a "voiding consequence" to whichever treatment you pursue.

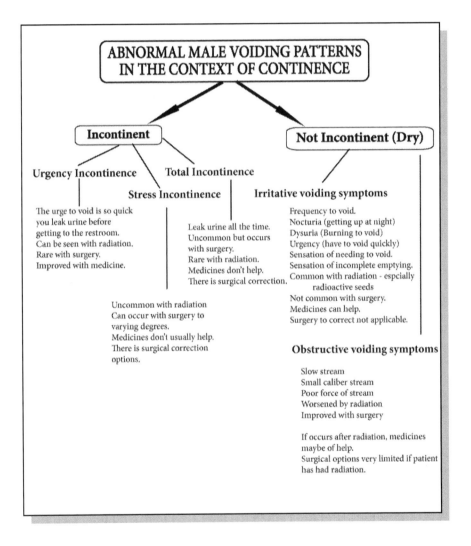

The quality of your erection - Sexual function

Pay me now or pay me later applies here too.

I remember the day as if it were yesterday. I had had my surgery on my wife's brother's birthday, May 10th, a Thursday. On June 6th, my wife's birthday, I called home to see if she would like me to pick something up for her birthday dinner. "I'd like Thai Dish; I really miss eating there." There used to be a Thai restaurant near our home that she loved, but it had moved to another location about 30 minutes from our house. The new location was inconvenient, and as a result we ate there infrequently. The round trip to this restaurant from my office and then to my home I figured would be about 40 minutes, and probably a good time to try taking a sex pill to see if I could "fire this baby up." Most of the pills have about a 30-minute window before they take effect. So as I am finishing up seeing patients for that afternoon, I get a sample pack from the drug cabinet and take one. By the time I had placed the to-go order and was in the car to pick it up, about 30 minutes had passed. Since I was still wearing a condom catheter because of the incontinence, I decided to shake the tubing that connects the bag to the condom and see if, on the way to Thai Dish, anything "perked up." There was a fair amount of anxiety associated with this test because of the chance that the surgery had messed up the nerves responsible for erections. It was a big deal to me as it is to all men treated for prostate cancer. I determined that there was life down there. It was not much, but the fact that I had any response at all indicated to me that, at a minimum, at least some of the nerves had been spared. I pranced into and out of Thai Dish and played the Beatles as loud as my CD player would allow with the windows down all the way home. (I love loud music in the car with the windows down.) When I got home with the food, my wife asked, "John, did you have a good day?" "Yes," I said, "It turned out to be a very nice day." June 6th is historically known as D-Day, but for me it's E-Day. In time, as the degree of my incontinence decreased and I was able to go to back to a diaper, I was very content and actually felt lucky to be "dry with a diaper, potent with a pill."

> ## *Dry with a diaper-Potent with a pill.*

The nerves necessary for erections run along the posterior lateral aspect of the prostate and for this reason are negatively affected by any cancer treatment of the prostate. With radiation the nerves are damaged by the deleterious effect of the radiation; with surgery the nerves are injured in the process of removing the prostate. The Walsh nerve-sparing prostatectomy revolutionized the surgical removal of the prostate. This technique allows for the prostate to be removed without damaging these nerves, if the procedure is performed properly and if the anatomic location of the nerves allows sparing them.

If you are impotent or have poor erectile function, then post-treatment function should not be a factor in your decision. You can take this issue off the table. You would be surprised by how many patients will choose a particular form of therapy because of their concern regarding impotence even though they are unable to get an erection pretreatment.

The biggest factor in determining whether or not you will be potent after either treatment has a lot to do with your pretreatment erectile function. If your level of performance is a 10, you are on the young side for having prostate cancer, and you don't have other medical problems or take any medicines, you will have a much better chance of preserving erections than an older man on medicines that rates his function at 5. This is true for all forms of therapy.

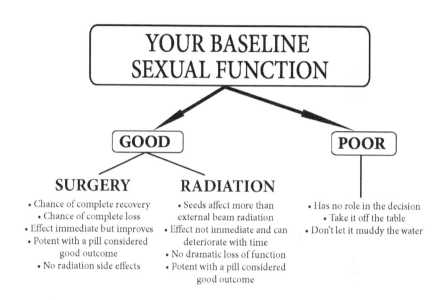

Surgery

Pay me now

I performed a prostatectomy on a 53-year-old patient for whom sexual function was very important. I had made clear to him on numerous occasions that he could possibly be impotent after the surgery. I actually was trying to talk him out of me doing his surgery because he was a friend, and I knew how important his sex life was to him. I did not want the baggage of any post-operative sexual issues, influencing our friendship. He made clear to me that, although sexual function was very important to him, he felt that because of his young age, the need to have the prostate removed was more important. The evening after his surgery I stopped by his room to check on him. His first question was, "How much blood did I lose?" His second question was, "Can you bring by a sample of one of those sex pills tomorrow morning? I want to see if I have any function." The next morning as requested I brought him a sample of one the popular brands of "sex pills," and, as it turned out, he was doing well and went home that day. I called him at home that evening to see how things were going. "John, I took that pill you gave me, I think I am going to be alright, I have already had an erection." When I say the issue of erectile function is very important to some, this is what I mean.

> This guy was less than 24 hours out from major surgery, had a catheter in his bladder and was taking medicines to see if he could get an erection! How or what he did to come to his happy conclusion I did not ask.

The best-case scenario for preserving erectile function in a healthy male with no medical problems, taking no medications, and normal sexual function pretreatment is a properly performed removal of the prostate. After surgery, if the nerves are spared and only bruised, your erectile function takes an initial hit, but the function will improve from the time of surgery for up to one year or longer, often to pretreatment levels. (I was fortunate in that this was the case for me.) This differs dramatically from radiation, in which baseline function is not affected initially but deteriorates to an unknown level over time and stays at that level. I said "best case scenario" because if you have surgery and the nerves are not spared, you have a greater risk of dramatic and immediate loss of function that may or may not recover. In a lot of patients, it is the potential for this dramatic loss that drives their decision towards radiation, weighing this concern more heavily than the potential for the slow gradual loss associated with radiation. As mentioned earlier, a properly performed Walsh nerve-sparing prostatectomy will usually prevent the scenario of the dramatic, non-recoverable loss of potency. The bet that the patient makes here, one that has to be considered in the decision formula, is shown in the following: There is a higher risk of complete loss of erections but higher chance of complete recovery with surgery. With radiation it is unlikely that your erections will stay as good as they are, however, you are betting that there will not be complete loss and that the deterioration will be slow and minimal. To some, this is a better scenario than the risk of complete loss if the nerves for whatever reason are not spared at the time of surgical removal.

The fluid in the ejaculate of a male comes from the seminal vesicles, prostate, and the testicles by way of the vas deferens. At the time of a prostatectomy the vas deferens is transected, and the prostate and seminal vesicles are removed; this results in eliminating all of the fluid that would normally be present at the time of ejaculation. The external sphincter (the feel-good muscle), which is left intact, is responsible for the climax associated with sexual activity. So, after the prostate is removed you will continue to have a climax but no fluid. For some patients, the quality and character of the climax are altered. What it will be like for you is not predictable.

Radiation

Pay me later

If your erectile function is good and you have radiation, the negative effect of the radiation on the nerves will not be immediate. Your erectile function eventually will take a hit over time, and the level of function that you end up with varies based on your pretreatment erectile function and your medical health. If you are on medicines for other conditions, particularly high blood pressure, diabetes, or heart disease, these will also play a role in your ultimate level of sexual function. The time period in which the negative effect of the radiation has had its full influence varies from patient to patient and can't be predicted. Just as with surgery, there are treatments available to treat the negative effect of radiation on your erectile function. External beam therapy has less effect on sexual function than brachytherapy. Brachytherapy, particularly if the radiation therapist places more seeds laterally (because the location of the cancer on the biopsy report is near the capsule), can affect sexual function more profoundly than external beam. As you recall, the nerves that are responsible for erections are at the back, lateral sides of the prostate. If the radioactive seeds are placed in this area to kill cancer cells, one can understand why this would negatively affect the nerves in that area and subsequently result in the loss of sexual function with time. If the radiation therapist purposely tries not to put seeds in this area to lessen the effect on sexual function, then he is compromising the treatment of the cancer. When given the choice, making sure there is an adequate radiation dose in a particular area of the prostate takes precedence over salvaging erectile function. Obviously, if seeds and external beam are utilized, this combination would have a more deleterious effect on the nerves, and hence sexual function, than either of the forms of radiation alone.

As a note, the patients that I see who have radiation and ultimately experience erection difficulties are often surprised by it. Many have chosen radiation because they believed that their erectile function had a better chance of salvage with radiation than surgery. This is not is not always the case, but I hear it often. To summarize: Surgery has a higher chance of complete loss of sexual function if the nerves are damaged, but a better chance of complete recovery if the nerves are spared. Radiation has a very low likelihood of early complete loss of sexual function, but the chance of deterioration with time to an unknown level. In both cases erectile function takes a hit but in different time frames, for different reasons, and ending with an unpredictable final level of function. The pearl here is that you have heard about the potential for loss of sexual function with surgery, so be sure to explore the potential for loss of sexual function with radiation and factor that into your ultimate decision.

Comparing the two

- When the nerves are damaged by radiation they do not regenerate; whatever you are left with after radiation is what you get. The negative effect on erections from radiation evolves with time. Surgery affects erections early on and then improves if nerves are spared at the time of the prostatectomy.

- If you are choosing radiation because you feel or have been told that you will have a better chance at maintaining your current level of sexual function, you may be making a treatment decision on the wrong premise. Again, age, medical health, baseline function and the specifics of which treatment you are going to have influence post treatment function. Both surgery and radiation can negatively impact your sexual function.

• External beam radiation has less of an effect on erectile function than seeds. The combination of seeds and external beam radiation has more effect on erectile dysfunction than seeds alone.

• The effects of radiation on the body and the nerves responsible for erectile function can evolve over years and to what degree it will affect you cannot be predicted.

• With surgery you have a greater chance of complete loss of sexual function, but if the nerves are appropriately spared, you have a better chance of returning to normal function with the added benefit of having had no radiation. A patient has a less chance of dramatic loss of function after treatment with radiation.

• Sexual function deterioration caused by either radiation or surgery can often be corrected with medication and other treatments currently available.

• For oral medicines to correct radiation or surgical induced sexual dysfunction, there has to be some degree of nerve function and partial erection. Intracorporal injections of vasoactive drugs bypass the need for the nerves and hence a patient can get an erection if the nerves are completely damaged by either therapy. This is important in that erectile dysfunction post therapy is very treatable, albeit in a way that is not, "like it used to be."

• After radiation, your ejaculate (semen) will be diminished or absent from the effect of the radiation "drying up" the prostate gland. The prostate produces most of the fluid in the ejaculate so it makes sense that this will be affected.

• After surgery, you will have no ejaculate. The prostate is gone, and the tubes that carry the sperm from the testicles (the vas deferens) are tied off at the time of removing the prostate.

Lifestyle-driven - *Ease of treatment is your priority*

Be careful not to choose short-term gratification over long-term gain. (My mother's most repeated "motherism" and the one most responsible for me going to and getting through medical school; this concept should be considered in, and applied to, your decision as well.)

The reason radiation therapy, and particularly seeds, appealed to me was because the time out of work required for this form of treatment is minimal. Who wants to have surgery and go through all that entails if there is an easier route and the results are about the same? This is a very common first impression that many patients have after being informed that they have prostate cancer, and the reason many patients choose radiation. Seed therapy makes for an easy sell on the surface. An incision, a catheter, and the certainty of at least some post-operative incontinence for an undetermined period of time after surgery make the non-surgical options attractive. Not many people outside of my profession realize this, but as a physician, I make income only if I am working. I am paid well, but if I am not physically seeing patients, no income is generated. Additionally, my responsibility for overhead, which includes my office and its attendant expenses, supplies, and employees, continues. In terms of the potential deleterious effect it would have on me financially, having surgery was a big deal. A major complication that prevented me from getting back to work in a reasonable time would have been financially devastating to me, and this complicated my situation and decision-making process. The benefits of surgery from a purely medical standpoint had to outweigh the disadvantage of the time away from work and the benefits and ease of radiation. I decided upon surgery for several reasons pertinent only to me, and I felt the medical and long-term benefits of surgery justified that decision. You too will have to do the same assessment, but your decision will be peculiar to your situation and one that you feel is best for you.

If working is important and necessary for you, and missing work a hardship, then radiation, particularly seed therapy, will be appealing to you. If time away from work or play is your driving issue, you will reason that the cure rates are very similar in radiation and surgery, that the difference in side effects is six of one and a half a dozen of the other, and you'll go with the treatment that impacts your life the least. A lot of patients base their decision on this alone, and, in my opinion, it is a valid rationalization if the other issues we have discussed have been considered and vetted. Work and time out from work have major roles to play in the decision, and certainly more so in the patients diagnosed during their working years. This issue is not as important to someone older or retired, for whom work and time off from work does not factor as prominently. For instance, a teacher with the summer off will weigh the work issue less than the person who is self-employed, for whom being out of work for a period of time would be very costly to him and his family. In a similar way, many patients have family or social restraints that preclude surgical removal and its attendant down-time. The radiation options impact daily life less and might be favored for this reason. An example here is the patient who has a family member that needs his assistance throughout the day, and who might choose radiation because he can continue with his home obligations while undergoing treatment.

Internet/family/friends – *Apples to apples/Prostates to prostates*

A little knowledge – Don't get too cute with what you've learned from your research; there is no reason to "go it alone" in making your decision.

> ## Don't be clever by half.

*On one particular occasion (however it has happened countless times) I had just told a patient that his biopsy showed cancer. I began to lay out an overview of the options and happened to start with surgery. Before I could continue, the patient told me, "My brother has a friend who has prostate cancer, and he did radiation because a doctor told him that if he had surgery he'd be impotent and that surgery lets air get to the prostate and will make it spread. My brother **and** his friend told me to steer clear of* *surgery." Now, normally I will take a deep breath and slowly explain the pros and cons of both radiation and surgery and the concept of apples to apples, but sometimes I have a little fun showcasing the folly of how some patients will place so much credence on something someone has told them. On this occasion I said, "Mr. Jones, thank you for sharing that with me. What type of work does your brother do?" "He sells insurance." "Thank you. And what type of work does your brother's friend do?" "I think he builds houses." I then said," Okay. Based on what you have told me, this is what I'd recommend for **your** cancer. My advice to you would be for you to do what your brother said his friend was told by his doctor about your brother's friend's cancer. Do you have any other questions for me?"*

Once you know you have prostate cancer and a few people find out about it, you'll begin to think that almost everybody and their brother has or has had prostate cancer. "It's like people with prostate cancer came out of the woodwork," I've been told often. Although I advise patients to learn as much as possible about prostate cancer treatment options from the internet and to seek the counsel of friends and family, you have to be careful. You have previously read about all the factors that go into this decision. To base a decision on what a friend did or what "his doctor" him told without knowing the specifics is truly unreliable and frankly foolish. It is reasonable to consider radiation or surgery more favorably if a friend had it done and did well, but hopefully this book will allow you to compare apples to apples. Ask intelligently, "What was your Gleason's score, baseline erectile function, how old are you, what is your current voiding pattern and what are your other medical conditions?" If his answers demonstrate parameters that are different from yours, and they probably will, then "his treatment" may be totally wrong for you. An example that comes to mind is a patient of mine who was recently diagnosed with prostate cancer and told by a friend at church that he should have "the robot" surgery. The patient had significant lung disease because of a longstanding smoking history and was clearly not a candidate for the four-hour anesthesia required for that procedure. The patient nevertheless spent a day going to Atlanta for an appointment with the robotic surgeon only to be told that he was not a candidate for it because of his lung disease. No harm was done in this futile exercise, but certainly this patient's time could have been better spent with his urologist fashioning a treatment plan suitable to his underlying medical problem pertaining to his lungs. In this patient's case, external beam radiation with no anesthesia required or seed therapy under regional anesthesia would be most reasonable for him, i.e. his lung condition limits his treatment options, ruling out surgical removal of the prostate. Speak to your friends and family who have had cancer from the standpoint of a knowledgeable understanding of your particular situation. Always think apples to apples; if the person advising surgery is 50 and in good health and you are 70 and have lung disease, keep that in mind. Utilize the internet with the above caveats, and then use the information gleaned to better question your friends, urologist, or radiation therapist. It is not unusual for a patient to be in the exam room with his board-certified urologist with a stack of papers printed off the internet in his lap, having made his decision without asking for any advice. This happens to me usually on the visit after the diagnosis of cancer has been made known, and the patient is returning for the results of the staging work-up. Once I give the good news that there is no obvious spread of the cancer beyond the prostate, he then pronounces his decision without any further consultation. (Anything I might say contrary to his "well thought-out" decision would be perceived as trying to talk him out of it, and I prefer not doing that with patients.)

My brother Bob once sold used cars. It was always humorous to him how customers would come in with cost comparisons that had been obtained from either another dealership or the internet. The customer, in my brother's view, almost always had a false sense of security about their knowledge of the worth of their used car or their ability to negotiate. My brother related to me an adage well known in the car business that relates not only to a used car customer but also to a "little knowledge" type of patient. My brother would pose this question to me: "John, if you're betting between a salesman who does what he does for a living 365 days a year and Joe Blow, the customer, who buys a car once every five years, who do you think will win?" The tangential analogy here is that it is foolhardy to do research on your own and make your mind up without filtering your research through the prism of a specialist who deals with this disease on a daily basis. Many patients rightfully ask, "You do this all the time, what would you advise?" It is surprising, however, how often it occurs that after a patient is informed of the diagnosis, he does some research or is impressed with a brochure that he got in the mail and doesn't come back to the urologist for further consultation. In this type of patient, two factors are in play. They have wrongly assumed that they already understand all the nuances of the disease and the treatments, and they feel that the urologic surgeon is going to recommend surgery. This patient's thinking is that because the urologist is a "if all you have is a hammer, the whole world is a nail" type of person, there is no reason to go back. Because the urologist is the one that does the biopsy, it will be the urologist that tells you that you have cancer and in turn becomes the gateway to the decision-making process. To assume that the urologist will guide you exclusively to surgery in most cases is in error. The reason I can tell you this with confidence is that the potential for life-altering changes in your erectile function and voiding pattern is real. Most urologists want the decision to be made by the patient and his family, and for the right reason, because if a complication does occur, there is no second-guessing about the surgery having been coerced. (If a patient has a problem with surgery, he blames the surgeon, but if he has a problem with radiation, he blames the radiation. That's a big difference.) I will usually give the patient the results of the biopsy and an overview of the treatment options with some informative literature on one visit, and after a week or so, further discuss options on another visit. I will work through the "who are you" with them and family members, and together we gravitate to a decision based on all of the factors. Neither I, nor most urologists, want to do surgery on a patient who is uncertain which treatment is best for him. In this scenario, we give the patient more time and often suggest a second opinion with a radiation therapist. I have had patients tell me immediately after I informed them of the positive biopsy, "I can tell you this; I ain't gonna let you cut on me." There is not a lot you can do for a patient like this, and there is no reason to labor over trying to change his mind. His feelings reflect a preconceived notion that the doctor does not have the best interest of the patient in mind. If you have underlying suspicions or mistrust regarding your doctor, you should get another doctor. **Also, it is rarely a bad idea to get a second opinion, and my advice is to get it with a radiation therapist, not another urologist.** You already have the surgeon's perspective; I don't think much will be gleaned from another urologist. Do your research, and then filter what you have learned through your doctors to arrive at a decision that is best for you. Don't be a one-issue patient if you can help it.

When a patient lets "a little knowledge" get mixed in with "clever by half," he ends up making the wrong decision.

A wise man takes counsel of his friends...and his urologist.

> ### Another "motherism"- A wise man doesn't need advice, a fool won't take it.

Misconceptions and half-truths – *Don't let "a little knowledge" get you.*

*"How did you end up choosing cryotherapy, Mr. Bolton?" I asked a patient when he returned for follow-up for his prostate cancer. He represented yet another patient in whom I had diagnosed prostate cancer and, without consulting me, had arranged to have his treatment done elsewhere and return for me to keep a check on the cancer. In this instance the patient had had cryosurgery in the Atlanta area. A friend of his had told him that cryosurgery had the highest rate of cure and the least chance of impotency. I did not have the heart to tell him that what he'd been told was not accurate and that impotence is **more** likely after cryosurgery when compared to other treatment modalities. How could a successful businessman pursue a treatment without at least running his ideas past his urologist or some other caregiver? I am not opposed to the decision he made; however it is breathtaking how often patients will make such a serious decision based on inaccurate information.*

Had he asked my opinion on cryosurgery I would have told him it was a reasonable choice, particularly if his biopsy report was favorable, if his gland was small in size, and if the increased risk of impotence were acceptable to him. I would have mentioned that one advantage of cryosurgery is that if the cancer does come back you can do cryosurgery a second time. I would have made it clear to him that I did not "have a dog in this fight," and that it doesn't upset or disappoint me if a patient chooses a treatment other than surgery. Patients should use their physicians like one should use an attorney: sap them for all the information and advice you can, and then work on your decision. I see this patient's behavior often, and I believe that some patients get it in their head that they will get a more unbiased answer from a friend who has had a particular procedure than they would from the doctor. They also place too much weight on their research. It reminds me of my investments. I have read extensively on investing, but have learned the hard way that, as when buying a used car, my expertise cannot compare to the person that does it every day for a living. On this particular visit with this patient, he told me, "I can't believe that it took away my sex life like that; I have no function at all, and why didn't they tell me that this would happen?" Being new and fancy, done in a big town, and having a nice brochure does not necessarily make something a good choice. When I was a resident I would moonlight working in an emergency room for extra money on weekends in the small town of Millen, Georgia, about an hour's drive from Augusta, Georgia. There was a seasoned physician there that I would consult from time to time about various patients I saw in the emergency room. When I would occasionally suggest that the patient might be better served being seen in Augusta at the Medical College, he would say sarcastically, "Oh yes, Doctor, send him to the bright lights of Augusta he'll do so much better

*there." Don't let the "bright lights" blind your decision-making
process.*

Misconceptions are secondary areas of concern in making your
decision. It would surprise you, however, just how many patients
base what they do on what a friend or family member has done or
information that they heard from others. I would advise that you
read and listen to others, but read and listen intelligently and
discerningly. It is unfortunate when a patient comes in for his
follow-up visit after having done his research and soul searching,
and the decision that has been arrived at is based on the wrong
information. It might be an apple to orange fact from a family
member, something suggested by an ad found on the internet,
something received in the mail, or misconceptions regarding
surgery or radiation. The following are misconceptions that I hear
commonly and, surprisingly, one or more of these I have seen used
as the basis for a patient's decision. You will be able to tell by the
nature of each how it could influence choosing for or against a
particular treatment.

- *Everyone who has surgery will leak urine.*

- *Radiation will "burn you."*

- *Impotence is always less common when treated with
radiation.*

- *Allowing air to touch the cancer will make it spread.*

- *All prostate cancers are slow-growing.*

- *All prostate cancers are the same.*

- *High dose herbs will help.*

- *Sticking holes in the prostate to place radioactive seeds will spread the cancer.*

- *Most people die "with it", not "of it."* True to a degree, but this should not drive the decision. Remember to utilize the particulars of the biopsy, exam, and PSA to help you determine the aggressiveness of your cancer.

- *Prostate cancer is a disease of "old" men.* I removed a prostate full of cancer in a 39-year-old man incidentally found to have an elevated PSA on a work physical.

- *A prostate biopsy is terribly painful.*

- *A prostate biopsy will spread the cancer.*

- *The PSA determination is unreliable and not helpful.* There is a high false positive rate with the PSA (elevated, but not because of cancer), true, but all agree that the PSA has allowed for early detection of prostate cancer and has saved lives.

- *Surgery always "cuts the nerves" and causes impotence.*

- *All surgeons want to do is cut and will always*

recommend surgery.

• *Robotic removal prostatectomy is better than the traditional open method.* The cure rates are no better with robotic and the chances of impotency and incontinence are similar. I have had patients brag to me about having the "robot done" and how well it went, but when I inquire whether they were "dry and potent" they shake their head and say, "I'm having problems there." Know the pros and cons of robotic removal discussed elsewhere this book. Robotic still means removing the prostate; the surgical changes to your anatomy are exactly the same as the open method, and you'll have to deal with exactly the same issues as a result of that. The length of stay in the hospital and blood loss is reduced with the robotic removal. Depending on your community, you may have to travel out of town to have it done, and at times acceptance of insurance by the surgeon is an issue. Open removal by a experienced surgeon probably trumps robotic removal by an inexperienced surgeon. Consider all the factors in your decision. Also remember that there are short-term medical issues (hospital stay) and long-term urological issues (incontinence, erectile function, and cure) to consider. At this point its biggest advantage addresses the short-term issues.

• *If you remove the prostate surgically and it's out of your body, you're cured right?* Not if there is a small amount of cancer outside the prostate prior to its removal.

- *"I recently had a colonoscopy; that would have checked the prostate wouldn't it?"* The colon is a separate organ and the prostate is not checked by that procedure.

- *I'm 60; don't most men my age have prostate cancer anyway? Why check for it?* Around forty percent of autopsied men who are 60 have pathological evidence of prostate cancer. This doesn't mean it would be clinically evident, and this statistic doesn't take into account the percentage of those glands that are high Gleason's grade. In addition, you have to have a biopsy to see if you have prostate cancer as well as to determine the volume and grade (Gleason's score). In general, if prostate cancer is detected on a prostate biopsy, it is clinically significant; this is different than the autopsy evaluation of the prostate in which the entire gland is examined. "A little knowledge is a dangerous thing."

- *A bad life style causes prostate cancer.* Testosterone, which all men produce, contributes to prostate cancer. (A study of eunuch (no testicles) monks revealed no incidence of prostate cancer. Heredity, being of African descent, and consuming a high fat diet common to industrialized countries does contribute to prostate cancer.

- *My friend did well with a particular treatment so I will too.*

Misconceptions abound as well about the male that has prostate cancer. All of the half-truths that might impede the diagnosis in males are now attributed to the male that has it and has been treated. Let me explain. I was a bit different in how I handled the news that I had prostate cancer compared to most patients and probably differently from you. I did not tell many people; I had emotional difficulty telling my children and did not want it announced at church, like you hear so often during prayer concerns. I personally felt that I was dealing with the diagnosis of cancer fairly well, but that retelling it to others would be difficult for me. I have been that way all my life; my aunt Betsy once said to me, "It's a Davis family trait, John; your grandfather would cry at the drop of a hat." I had this fear of becoming emotional in telling my children the news, so I delayed doing anything for several weeks and finally decided I'd send an email. I used as the subject line, "dad's got a new gig." In my email I rambled on and only implied that I had cancer ("the biopsy showed something"), but reassured them that I would be O.K. It was a very difficult time for me; I was more concerned about how they would feel about their dad having cancer than the threat that I would not do well. As I have previously mentioned, I kept having the sensation and feeling that somehow I had let all of my family down. When they called to ask what in the world I was talking about in my cryptic email, my wife did all the explaining. For about a month I did not answer the phone; the thought of telling one of my children that I had cancer was something I just could not do. It took weeks before I could talk of it without my eyes welling up. It was embarrassing. My wife was absolutely beautiful and strong through this, explaining "my situation" to all family members that would call inquiring about me as if I were not home, although I'd be there next to her in our den. I did tell a female friend, with whom I teach youth Sunday school (I have taught youth Sunday school at my church for about 20 years) about a month or so after my diagnosis. She had had breast cancer, and I felt almost guilty that I had not told her. Once *she knew, she would ask each Sunday when was I going to do something about the cancer. After about two months of this questioning each Sunday, she exasperatedly said to me in the parking lot outside the church, **"John, go get your prostate cancer treated; you'll have sex again!"** I thought it was an odd remark at the time, but I suppose she thought my delay in making a decision was a "male thing." In retrospect there may have been some truth and intuition in her observation, a "woman thing." This remark then began a new era of issues for me surrounding the misconceptions of others in their understanding of what happens to you when you've been treated for prostate cancer. It is a reverse misconception, so to speak, not about the male's understanding of prostate cancer, but others' misconceptions about someone who has been treated. I began to wonder, are she and others thinking that I will be impotent and incontinent; is this how others will view me in the future? As hard as the decision is, this added element, particularly in a relatively young man, adds to the stress of dealing with the purely medical issues of prostate cancer. This disease and associated treatment options are unusual in that concerns regarding potency and incontinence issues are often moved to the forefront and cure is placed on the back burner. In many ways the treatment of prostate cancer is a "male mastectomy." In a female there is the emotional trauma of having breast cancer and treatments that can disfigure the body; in the male there is no disfiguration that you can see, but treatment of the prostate affects the quality of how you void and achieve erections. There is also the constant awareness that the cancer may not have been cured and "come back." This does somewhat eat at your maleness, and knowledge of these risks complicates the decision.*

In many ways the treatment of prostate cancer, and its attendant emotional and physical consequences, parallels a woman's journey with breast cancer.

McHugh Decision Worksheet – *Have you learned enough about yourself and your prostate cancer to answer these questions intelligently?*

Evaluate the "Who are you" issues, your cancer specifics, and the risks and benefits of the treatments; then fill out this worksheet. If you score mostly 1's and 2's, you are a radiation type; mostly 4's and 5's, you may be a surgery type; mostly 3's, then you are probably undecided. Use the insight gleaned here in addition to your other research to help you reach your decision. At the end of the worksheet are caveats related to each question, previously referenced in this book, which should be considered and well thought out in each of your answers. **(A printable PDF download of this worksheet can be found under "Helpful Links" at theprostatedecision.com.)**

> Your "Decision" is more complicated than just doing what someone you know did.

1. How important is it to have other options for treatment if your PSA begins to rise after surgery or radiation?				
Not important	Minimally important	Somewhat important	Important	Very important
1	2	3	4	5

2. Does the need for an incision, a catheter, and the risk of incontinence deter you from surgical removal?				
Yes - very much	Yes	Probably	Probably not - other factors more important	Not a factor - other issues drive my decision
1	2	3	4	5

3. Which most closely describes your biopsy and PSA?

Micro-focus on one side Gleason's 5-6 PSA normal or mildly elevated	Small volume on one side Gleason's 6 PSA normal or mildly elevated	Small volume on both sides Gleason's 6 PSA between 4-10	Moderate volume on both sides Gleason's 6-7 PSA between 4-10	High volume on both sides Gleason's 7 or higher PSA over 10
1	2	3	4	5

4. How would you describe your urinary stream?

Completely normal, on no prostate meds	Minimal obstructive voiding symptoms	Mild symptoms, on prostate medication	Off-and-on slow stream, small caliber of urinary stream	Slow, with small force and caliber of urinary stream
1	2	3	4	5

5. Which most closely matches your health and age?

Marginal health, over 70 years of age	Good health, over 70 years of age	Marginal health, aged 60-70	Good health, 40-65 years of age	Excellent health, 40-65 years of age
1	2	3	4	5

6. Above all other issues, the most aggressive method to treat your cancer is the one most important to you.

Definitely not most important factor.	Probably not most important issue	Undecided - other factors play a role	Yes	Very strongly yes
1	2	3	4	5

7. Do you think surgical removal or radiation gives you a better chance of preserving sexual function long term?

Definitely radiation	Radiation	About the same	Surgery	Definitely surgery
1	2	3	4	5

8. Which treatment do you feel is most likely to cure you of your prostate cancer?				
Radioactive seeds and external beam radiation.	Probably radiation	Don't know - about the same.	Probably surgical removal	Surgical removal of the prostate
1	2	3	4	5

9. How important is the ease of treatment, limited time out of work, and impact on lifestyle to you?				
Most important factor in my decision	Important - has large role in my decision	Somewhat important - other issues also factor	Not a primary factor in my decision	Ease of treatment has no role at all in my decision
1	2	3	4	5

10. What method of treatment would you choose if it were based solely on your personal research, the wishes of your family, and your interviews of friends who have been treated for prostate cancer?				
Radiation	Probably radiation	Don't know	Probably surgical removal	Surgical removal
1	2	3	4	5

Important points to consider and understand in answering each question.

1. You can do full course external beam radiation after surgical removal if there is a later rise in your PSA. If you have radiation first and your PSA rises, indicating a return of your cancer, you have limited options for surgical intervention to treat the cancer or any of the side effects of radiation, i.e. obstructive voiding symptoms.

2. This question hits at the ease of therapy issue. Radiation with seeds is an outpatient, 90-minute procedure with anesthesia and wearing a catheter usually for only one day. Surgery is associated with more risks, longer hospital stay, longer need for a catheter, and an incision or incisions depending on the method chosen to remove the prostate. If ease of therapy is your main focus, this is hands down in favor of radiation. External beam therapy is inconvenient in terms of the number of trips required for treatment but is simple to do with minimal treatment risks.

3.   The characteristics of your biopsy give you insight as to the aggressiveness of your cancer. I believe that surgical removal is the most aggressive form of treatment for prostate cancer. (Your radiation therapist may disagree, ask him or her for yourself and get their view.) If your biopsy indicates aggressive disease, you should be thinking more about aggressive therapy. If your biopsy suggests a less aggressive cancer, you may opt for the less aggressive therapy, radiation or cryotherapy, in hopes of having both a curative result and ease of treatment.

4.   If you are having problems with a slow stream, this should heavily influence your decision. You now know that surgical removal will help this symptom, which is most likely unrelated to your cancer and related just to the natural enlargement of the prostate commonly seen in males as they age. You also realize that radiation will make this symptom worse, and if you are adamant about pursuing radiation as your treatment of choice, a procedure to correct it must be done before radiation because surgical correction after radiation is fraught with difficulties. (It is better to cure at the beginning rather than the end.)

5.   It all starts with good health; if you don't have it you will not be a candidate for surgical removal and possibly not a candidate for seeds, as seed implantation also requires anesthesia. If you are in good health but in your mid-70s, then your years at risk come into play and you may choose a less aggressive therapy, potentially leaning toward radiation, particularly external beam. If the cancer

does reoccur, your age or other medical problems may make it irrelevant. Good health and young physiologic age indicate an extended years-at-risk profile and favor a more aggressive therapy. Marginal health and limited years at risk favor a less aggressive therapy.

6. This stresses the point that a patient needs to declare to himself what he feels is most important to him regarding treatment. It will either be cure, and what he feels is the most aggressive form of therapy will be the driving factor, or a blend of ease of treatment with an acceptable cure rate. The cure-only patient, like I was, is a "Damn the torpedoes - I want it out!" type. If other factors rule your thought process, you may opt for a less aggressive route in an attempt to "have your cake and eat it too."

7. This is a trick question, but obviously if preserving sexual function is important to you, you really need to know the caveats here. In a nutshell, surgical removal has more risk of the complete dramatic loss of sexual function if the nerves are severed at the time of the prostatectomy. You now know, however, that with a properly performed Walsh Nerve Sparing Prostatectomy and some luck, your nerves will be spared and your erectile function will be salvaged. If the nerves are spared, sexual function can return to your baseline. Surgery is big risk, big reward. Radiation will not result in the dramatic loss of sexual function, but you may see a deterioration of your erections over time to an undetermined level, even impotence. The reason this is a trick question is that sexual function takes a hit with either treatment, and when you consider all the factors and potential end points of the various treatments, this question is probably a wash and number 3 is the right answer. In my case, sexual function slowly improved over the course of a year to the point that I no longer need to take drugs for erections. Remember that I was relatively young and had no other medical problems at the time of my surgery. The degree to which sexual function is preserved with either of the treatments depends heavily on the pretreatment erectile function and general health of the patient.

8. Once you are told you have prostate cancer, you will begin weighing the risks against the benefits of the various treatment options. Some patients worry less about the risks than their general feeling of what is the most aggressive form of therapy and the one that they feel gives them the best shot at cure. In general, an aggressive mindset is a surgery type; someone who is weighing risks, benefits, and concerns about impact on lifestyle is generally a radiation type. (This is a rephrasing of question **6,** but this is so important. It is not wrong to heavily value the ease of a particular treatment, but it is imperative to see it for what it is: a decision that is not based solely on cure.) As I have mentioned earlier in this book, as cancers go, prostate cancer is somewhat unusual in this regard, which is probably related to two issues. The first is the misconception that *all* prostate cancers act in a benign fashion (Why kill a fly with a shotgun?), and the second is the fear of potential complications, namely incontinence and impotence.

9. This question clearly differentiates the surgical removal-type patient from the patient who wants what he feels is a good treatment, but equally values impact on lifestyle and ease of the treatment. The patient of the latter mindset will usually choose radiation, particularly seeds, as it is an outpatient procedure involving 20-30 puncture wounds to the perineum, one day with a catheter, and no incision.

10. I added this question to make the point that patients will often value what they have learned through their personal research and what other people they know have done more that what their urologist may advise. This is not necessarily a flawed approach, but hopefully the apples to apples and prostates to prostates evaluation will prevent a patient with very unfavorable biopsy parameters from choosing to do what his friend with very favorable parameters did. Also, remember that procedures have both short and long-term effects. You must be aware of both and factor each into your decision as well.

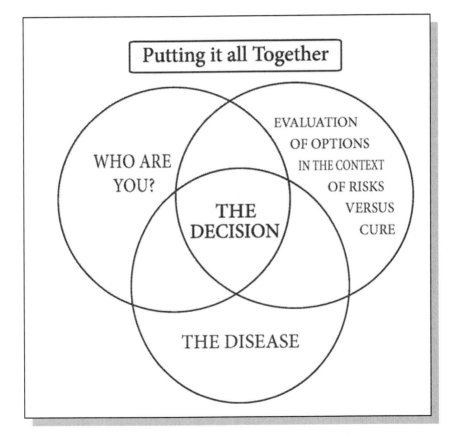

Part Three - Putting it all together - Methods for making the decision

Y ou now have the necessary foundation to make an informed decision about your prostate cancer. As seen in the illustration of interlacing circles, the main ingredients of the decision you now face involve three major areas. That is, your "who are you" factors, the risks weighed against the likelihood of cure, and the nature of your disease. Only you can assign the role each will play in your decision. What follows are some ways to evaluate what you now know in order to achieve closure in making your decision. I like to approach problems from different angles or from different perspectives and then match and compare the conclusions of each to reach a consensus, so to speak. You might even consider "thinking outside the box" scenarios. The methods listed are by no means the only ways this can be done; there may be a method that you have used for making other important decisions in your life. You can apply that method here; just plug in the pros and cons of the three major categories of this decision and see where it takes you. Again, take advantage of your family physician, radiation therapist, and urologist for any help they might offer in clarifying your decision. The following examples represent different angles to get at a decision; I have included my thought process in making my decision and thoughts on how you might make yours. My "Decision Cheat Sheet" addresses all the issues that have been previously discussed and offers a summarizing method.

Getting your priorities straight – *Paper covers rock*

Seeing the "big" picture

When I was a surgical intern in Augusta, Georgia in 1982, I was making rounds with a vascular surgery service. My group, which included interns, residents, nurses, and the attending physician, were standing around an unfortunate patient in the intensive care unit. This patient had tubes everywhere, was on many medicines, recently had had one leg removed from complications of diabetes, and now had developed some redness on a small area of his left arm. The chief resident began to spout off numerous options regarding what could be done, listed several diagnostic studies and lab tests that could be ordered, additional medications to institute, and then delineated the surgical options. All standing there including me were impressed by the litany of therapeutic options the chief resident delivered. After a pause, the attending physician said, "Harvey, have you ever seen the firefighters on T.V. fighting those fires in California?" The chief resident, somewhat puzzled, said, "Yes sir, I have." The attending continued in a prolonged Southern drawl, "You see them there with all that garb on and a backpack with a little hose shooting out a tiny stream of water at the base of one of those big California trees that is smoking, and all the while you see the forest fire behind them just raging out of control." The chief resident, who is just one step and weeks away from being a "real" doctor, and all the others assembled there just stood in silence trying to make sense of these obtuse words of wisdom and how they may be related to the patient we were all observing. After what seemed to be a long pause, with the attending physician peering at the patient and all of us peering at him, he said, "Harvey, let's just leave Mr. Johnson alone, why don't we?"

> ## It takes a smart doctor to know when a patient is dying.

A game you may have played when you were a kid, rock, paper, and scissors provides an analogy that can help with the decision. Let's say you have been recently diagnosed with prostate cancer and are otherwise in good health. This means that all of the available treatment options are open to you. You are in your early 60s, and sexual function is very important to you. You have symptoms of an enlarged prostate, unrelated to the cancer, which include slowing of your stream, getting up at night, and, if you have a beer, some urgency. The voiding symptoms do not require medicine but are such that you begin to notice them and are contemplating seeing your family doctor about them. You have seen a commercial or two about drugs for these symptoms and paid particular attention to them because they addressed your symptoms. In your research of the treatments and their effect on sexual function, you come to believe that the chance of preserving your erections is better with radiation. You have considered the caveats of each of the treatments on sexual function that have been previously discussed. *While it may not be clear that sexual preservation is better with radiation, the worsening of your voiding pattern after radiation is almost assured.* You may want to consider, keeping in mind the paper covers rock analogy, that radiation and its effect on voiding trumps the perceived advantage of radiation on sexual function versus that of surgery. In my opinion, if your sexual function is good and you have a properly performed prostatectomy, then the sexual function issue is a wash, and the decision should be made based on your anticipated voiding pattern after treatment. As discussed, radiation will likely worsen obstructive voiding symptoms, and surgery will improve them. The paper, which is to say voiding symptoms, covers the rock that is the impact on sexual function. If, after factoring in the impact on your family and job and the other risks of each treatment, you still feel radiation is best for you, then a procedure that improves your voiding pattern can be done before the anticipated radiation.

Now let's say you are the patient who from the get-go "wants it out." If he has other medical problems that would put him at risk for surgery, then the rock, his operative risk, crushes scissors, his desire for surgery, and he should consider radiation further. If a patient has a deep fear of total incontinence or dramatic loss of sexual function, although both have relatively low occurrences, then this fear trumps whatever other benefits he may feel removing the prostate has, and he would choose radiation. The ultimate decision has to be based on what is important to you, but with a foundation of knowledge of all the nuances of the various treatments. The decision scenarios and the "Decision Cheat Sheet" that follow balance what is important to you with the caveats of each treatment to help you arrive at the best decision for you, made for the right reasons.

You have good health and all options are open to you –
Evaluating your underlying health is an important part of the decision process.

When I review the chart outside of the patient's room and see that the biopsy performed several days before is positive for cancer, the first thing I do is look at the other medical problems. As I begin to lay out the options for the patient, it all starts with age and medical condition. If there is a problem with either of these, surgery is essentially taken off the table as an option. Remember this; no matter what treatment a patient chooses, he was given his diagnosis by a urologist. Around 50% of patients ultimately have radiation or some other treatment, which means that urologists are not pushing all of their patients toward surgery. By and large I feel most physicians, particularly urologists advising patients newly diagnosed with prostate cancer, are very conscientious regarding patient care and recommend what they feel is best and most appropriate for their patients.

The average surgical residency program lasts five years and begins after completing four years of medical school and four years of college.

> ## The first year of a surgical residency you are taught how to operate; the next four... when not to.

Obviously, good overall health is the first thing you should consider in choosing treatment. If you are inclined from your research that surgical removal is the best thing to cure the cancer, the risks associated with surgery because of your health may mean that radiation is a better option for you. (What's best for the cancer may not be the best thing for you.) The diagram which follows shows how your baseline health helps you to begin the process of deciding what you are going to do about your cancer:

How "who are you" issues and general health influence the decision

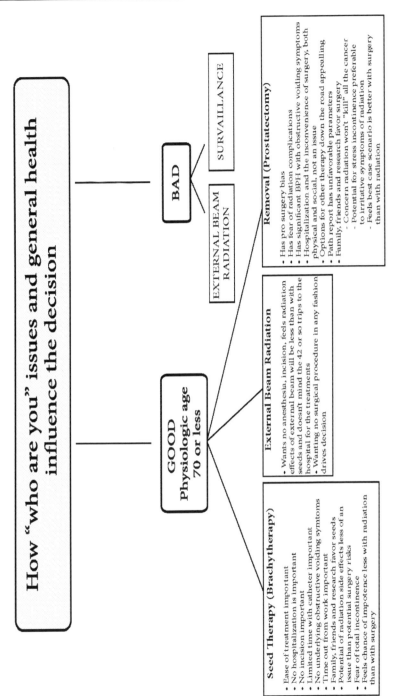

GOOD
Physiologic age
70 or less

BAD

EXTERNAL BEAM
RADIATION

SURVAILLANCE

Seed Therapy (Brachytherapy)

- Ease of treatment important
- No hospitalization is important
- No incision important
- Limited time with catheter important
- No underlying obstructive voiding symtoms important
- Time out from work important
- Family, friends and research favor seeds
- Potential of radiation side effects less of an issue than potential surgery risks
- Fear of total incontinence
- Feels chance of impotence less with radiation than with surgery

External Beam Radiation

- Wants no anesthesia, incision, feels radiation effects of external beam will be less than with seeds and doesn't mind the 42 or so trips to the hospital for the treatments
- Wanting no surgical procedure in any fashion drives decision

Removal (Prostatectomy)

- Has pro surgery bias
- Has fear of radiation complications
- Has significant BPH with obstructive voiding symptoms
- Hospitalization and the inconvenience of surgery, both physical and social, not an issue
- Options for other therapy down the road appealling
- Path report has unfavorable parameters
- Family, friends and research favor surgery
  - Concern radiation won't "kill" all the cancer
  - Potential for stress incontinence preferable to irritative symptoms of radiation
  - Feels best case scenario is better with surgery than with radiation

Evaluating the negatives- *Picking your poison*

Choosing "the lesser of two evils"

One technique that might help you to arrive at a decision is to look at all of the negative aspects of each of the treatments. On a sheet of paper, write out on one side the negatives of surgery and then on the other the negatives of radiation. Grade each as to how important it is to you and see which of the two treatments has the most negatives for you. I gave a copy of this book, in its early manuscript form, to a patient recently diagnosed with prostate cancer, and he returned a few weeks later to inform me that he had elected to have the prostate removed. When I asked why, and I often ask patients what was the most important factor in their decision, he said that he felt more comfortable with the potential risks of surgery than the potential risks of radiation. I had never had a patient put it quite that way, but if you feel the cure rates are similar, then you need to identify other issues to help you make a decision, and his method was certainly a reasonable way to get there. I might add that you must be knowledgeable of the risks of all the forms of therapy to use this method in helping you decide. From this standpoint, I feel the issues delineated in this book helped him and were beneficial to him in working through the process. There are other patients who feel that the risks of surgery and all it entails, a known, far outweigh the risks of radiation, an unknown. A patient who feels this way will choose radiation, a different conclusion, yet using the same logic. I see this all the time; it is very common with prostate cancer. My job and that of this book is to facilitate the patient in ultimately making a decision based on the facts most pertinent to him.

Best case/worse case scenarios- *Evaluating the potential outcome of your decision from different perspectives may be of help to you.*

Best case scenario- *A "trifecta"- cured, potent, and continent*

Another method you might employ is envisioning the best- or worst-case scenario for you with each treatment and see if one particular scenario overrides the other. The best-case scenario for surgery would be that you get through the surgery without any intra-operative complications, your sexual function is preserved, you are continent within a reasonable amount of time, and the cancer proves to have been confined to the prostate in the final pathology report. By choosing surgery, you have the added benefit of your body not having any radiation and the associated risks therein. The best-case scenario for radiation is that you have no complications related to radiation in the short or long term, your sexual function is preserved, you are continent, and the cancer doesn't come back. In the best-case scenario evaluation looking at the long-term picture, it seems that one is better off with surgery because no radiation was used. One must consider, however, that this benefit comes at the cost of the inconvenience and other issues involved with surgery up front. One could make the argument that the inconvenience and pain related to surgery in the short term are more of a disadvantage than your body's potential for adverse radiation risks in the long term despite the ease of treatment. In this situation one then has to determine if the benefits of not receiving radiation trump the problems of an incision, catheter, and other surgical issues. Now you see how it gets complicated; each of the issues will be weighted differently by different patients.

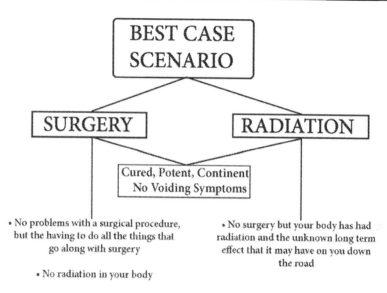

Worse case scenario

Now let's look at the worst-case scenarios. Obviously the worst-case scenario for surgery is a major intra-operative complication, which does not occur commonly but does occur. When you read the permit for a radical prostatectomy, and you should, you will see what I mean. Although the major complications don't occur often, blood loss, post-operative infections, deep vein thrombosis, and incontinence persisting for months after the catheter is taken out can all occur. Surgery may not spare the nerves, making you completely impotent. You might be totally incontinent or have unresolved stress incontinence after the catheter is removed. After all of this, your PSA might rise, requiring radiation and the potential of having complications related to that. I have had one patient die three days after a radical prostatectomy from a heart attack, unrelated to the surgery.

Worse case scenario paints quite a discouraging picture, making me wonder how in the world I chose surgery.

In regards to radiation, be sure to read the permit for this as well, as you may be surprised at the things that can happen with this treatment modality. Worst case scenario for radiation would be that your body is overly sensitive to radiation, and you get persistent diarrhea, worsening of undetected obstructive voiding symptoms, frequency, nocturia, urgency incontinence, and progressive loss of sexual function. If your situation progresses to the point you can't void, you have to wear a catheter until you can void, and that may take weeks to months. You and your urologist will be hesitant to pursue surgical procedures to relieve the obstruction because the risk of complications is high as a result of the tissues having been exposed to radiation. In this scenario, if the cancer returns, you have few options, as surgical removal after radiation is very difficult and fraught with complications. The rarer things might potentially occur: development of a fistula between the prostate and the rectum, hemorrhagic cystitis with intractable hematuria, bladder or rectal cancer years later as a result of the radiation. Radiation can continue to affect tissues many years after treatment and may influence subsequent surgical procedures that might be necessary for conditions of the abdomen. I have seen bleeding from the bladder, secondary to radiation cystitis, requiring endoscopic surgery or hyperbaric oxygen to correct, in patients who had radiation several years before.

> Read the informed consent (the permit) thoroughly for the treatment you choose. Ask your caregiver specific questions about anything that concerns you. The time to ask and understand is *before* your treatment.

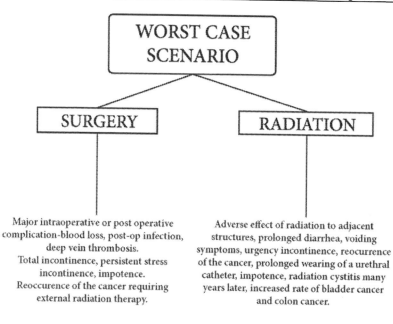

- *So, which worst-case scenario concerns you the most?*

- *Which scenario do you think is more likely to occur and which do you think you could deal with better if it did occur?*

- *Playing all the scenarios out, best case versus worst case, can you glean anything that helps you in the decision?*

- *Does the best of the best trump the worst of the worst?*

*It's not about doing **what** I did; it's about making your decision the **way** I did.*

How I made my decision

When I began the process of determining which treatment option was best for me, I had not yet formulated the "who are you" concept. However, I used it intuitively as I had when working through the options over the years with patients of mine. My general health was good; all options were open to me. Cure, ease of treatment, and time out of work concerns were the most important factors to me and vied for the most prominent role in my decision. *The risk of impotence and incontinence associated with surgical removal did not worry me as much as the complications and unknown future complications of radiation therapy.* Having performed hundreds of prostatectomies over the years and knowing how my patients have done with surgery gave me some degree of confidence about my favorable chances of retaining continence and potency. I also had confidence in the treatments necessary for the correction of these issues if they were to occur. In my practice, the patients who did well with surgery usually did very well, without the unknowns and potential downside of radiation. The inability for those who chose radiation, and had problems, to do anything other than take medicines was a big factor in my decision. At the time of my diagnosis, I had some underlying early symptoms of an enlarged prostate, mild frequency and some decreased caliber of my urinary stream, and I knew that radiation would most probably worsen that. The fact that I was 52 played a role as well. I knew that my years at risk, figuring that I would most probably live into my 70s, would be over 20 years. This made me gravitate heavily toward what I felt was the most aggressive way to deal with the cancer. My path report was favorable in terms of Gleason's score and volume, but my years at risk trumped this. The concern that cancer can return after radiation, not only because the cancer is outside the radiated field at the time of treatment, but because of the potential inability of radiation to kill the cancer, played a role here. Reoccurrence of prostate cancer after radiation, if it happens, usually happens five to eight years after treatment. The potential for inadequate placement with seeds heightened my concerns regarding my years at risk because those were probably longer than the average time to reoccurrence with radiation. In the end, my decision was driven by my belief that my best chance for cure was with surgery.

Summary of my decision – *Now, you work through the "who are you?" factors the same way, as I did, for your situation.*

- Underlying health was good; all the options were open to me.

- Cure vs. ease of treatment: cure was most important.

- Time out of work a concern but trumped by desire for most aggressive treatment.

- Unknown future effects of radiation concerned me more that the known potential complications of surgery. I felt that surgery was "cleaner" and that once I was over the surgery that would be it. (For me this has been the case.)

- Having other treatment options if the cancer came back was important to me.

- My underlying obstructive symptoms favored surgical removal, "killing two birds with one stone."

- My years at risk highly favored surgical removal.

- Being a surgeon, I just plain felt more comfortable with surgery.

- The influence of my friends and family was not a factor because I had my patients as models for how I might do with surgery. As a rule, they do quite well.

How you should make yours – *Now it's your turn*

Armed with the information in this book, you too can come to a decision about your cancer's treatment that you will become comfortable with. Begin with your general health and slowly work through which concerns trump others, and you will begin to narrow it down. The main point I'd like to make here is not to let your decision be one-dimensional (based on what a friend did, a commercial you saw, or a brochure you got in the mail). Ease of treatment, i.e. radiation, is a major concern for some; I explored that path as well. However, if you choose radiation because you feel there are fewer side effects, a better cure rate, or you are experiencing obstructive voiding symptoms, then you may be making an error. Have your radiation therapist thoroughly explain the negatives of radiation and be sure you are comfortable with his answers. If you have immediately gravitated to surgical removal, your health is marginal, and you are in your 70s, again you may be making the wrong decision. My advice is to explore all you know about your disease, your "who are you" factors, and discuss this with your health care providers to arrive at your decision.

I had a patient whom I had recently diagnosed with prostate cancer come into the office for a follow-up visit to review the results of his metastatic work up. After I told him, that to the best of our knowledge his cancer was confined to the prostate, he said, "Thank you, may I have my records? I have already made arrangements for radiation seed therapy." I did not make any attempt to dissuade him from his decision; I don't do that with patients. He and I stood up together and walked to the check-out area; we shook hands, and I told him that if I could ever be of any help to him, or if he had any voiding symptoms after the radiation, to let me know. He said thanks and walked to the exit, and I turned to begin seeing other patients. Just as he got to the door, he turned and said, "Dr. McHugh, am I making the right decision?" I smiled. "Step in here," I said, and we talked an additional 20 minutes in a room off of the check-out area. I complimented him on asking my advice and informed him of how often patients fail to do that. We talked about the pros and cons of both surgery and radiation, his "who are you" issues, and the latent effects of radiation. I don't speak negatively about radiation, but I do make sure that all the issues are understood and clarify that there is no free ride with either decision. I don't care what you decide; just make your decision for the right reasons and on the right information about the treatments. This particular patient ultimately chose surgery; however just as often, after a more thorough discussion the original decision, whether for surgery or radiation, holds and is the correct one. Again, do your research and then evaluate it with the input of your doctors. They are not there to trick or persuade you; we are all on the same team and have the same mutual goal, which is to try to do what is best for you. Complete the decision cheat sheet and see if it helps you in determining your inclinations. If you can intelligently answer all of the questions that follow, then this book has done its job, and tallying your responses after you've completed it will further aid you in clarifying your decision.

Decision Cheat Sheet – *Tally up all the factors to see where you stand.*

What follows represents a summary of the issues you should consider in making the decision. Some are redundant, but I think you will find, as I did, that evaluating an issue several ways will help you to hone your decision. For each category, circle the treatment that you feel is most suitable in your case and then tally your responses. You will be surprised by how helpful and comprehensive this exercise is, and at how knowledgeable you have become about the issues surrounding the decision.

P - Prostatectomy (You want the prostate removed, don't worry now about how.)

R -Radiation (Don't worry about which form, your radiation therapist will guide you.)

C - Cryosurgery

S - Surveillance (Remember this is an active process that entails serial PSAs and exams.)

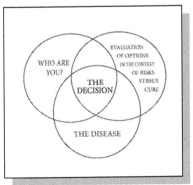

The Disease: Considering your disease (your PSA, rectal exam and path report), which treatment do you feel is best for you?	P	R	C	S

"Who are you" issues: For each category choose a treatment.

General health/Age and Years at risk: Does health limit you?	P	R	C	S
Bias: Do you have a preconceived notion of what to do?	P	R	C	S
Cure as main concern: Which do you feel has best chance of cure?	P	R	C	S

Risks are main concern:

Incontinence: Be sure to understand the different types.	P	R	C	S
Erectile function: Understand how each treatment affects it.	P	R	C	S
Short and long terms risks related to surgery vs. radiation.	P	R	C	S
Ease of treatment a priority: Is this important to you?	P	R	C	S
Family-friend-internet: What has your research gleaned?	P	R	C	S
Decision worksheet: Take it and put the result here.	P	R	C	S

	P	R	C	S
Evaluating the negatives: Which treatment has the least negatives?	P	R	C	S
Best case scenario: Which best outcome is most appealing to you?	P	R	C	S
Worse case scenario: Which bad outcome worries you least?	P	R	C	S
What does your "gut" tell you?	P	R	C	S
Which issue above drives your decision the most? Count your treatment choice for this issue as three when figuring your tally.	P	R	C	S

	P	R	C	S
Tally				

As in the decision worksheet, if there is a question that you do not understand all the ramifications of, go back to that part of the book to refresh your memory or consult other resources. This cheat sheet addresses the decision question from many angles and hopefully allows you to clarify your concerns and ultimately your decision. Well, how did you do? Tally your score, and hopefully your answers have given you a clear winner. If not, you have more work to do, and that's okay too. It took me three months to decide.

PDF of Decision Cheat Sheet at theprostatedecision.com

*Your evaluation of "who you are", knowledge of the specifics of **your** disease, and the assessment of risks vs. cure as they pertain to you, is the **key** to the right decision.*

Part Four - You've decided

T *he main focus of this book is to get you here, arriving at a decision either to have the prostate removed, use radiation, or pursue another treatment.* The hard part is done, but there are still smaller decisions to be made. In the case of surgery, it you must decide whether to have the prostate removed by the open method or by the robotic method. You may have additional issues regarding where and by whom the surgery will be done. In the case of radiation, whether you will be using seeds alone, external alone, or a combination of the two. Below is a brief delineation of the variations of the two major treatments and big concepts that will help you to further narrow your decision. A brief description of surveillance therapy and cryosurgery is included as well. Keep in mind that the first big decision is surgical removal or something else. If you don't choose surgical removal, then you have to decide from among the other options. Note that I use the term surgical removal, because, as previously mentioned, radioactive seeds and cryosurgery are surgical procedures requiring anesthesia but do not involve removal of the prostate.

You want it out – *Open vs. Robotic*

Now that you know you want the prostate removed, you need to decide between the conventional open surgical method and robotic removal. It is important to note that in both cases the prostate is removed, all of the dynamics related to its removal are the same, and the need for wearing a catheter exists for both. The major difference is that the open method involves a four-inch incision in the lower abdomen, and the robotic method utilizes seven small incisions or puncture wounds (needed for the laparoscopic instruments). *The robotic method is basically a laparoscopic procedure facilitated by the da Vinci robot.* Although there is no defined advantage of the robotic method over the open removal in terms of potency, incontinence, or cure rates; it does offer other advantages that do appeal to patients. Having said that, it makes sense to me that with less blood loss in addition to the magnification of the dissection that the robotic method provides, the likelihood of sparing the nerves and preserving sexual function may be enhanced. This assumes of course that the surgeon using the robot is experienced and skilled in the use of the robot and in the performance of the procedure. (A fool with a tool is still a fool.) With the robotic method, a one-night hospital stay is very common, blood loss is often times reduced, and patients usually tolerate the seven small incisions better than the one larger incision. Robotic removal would be a much easier decision and a slam-dunk option if it were not for the need for a catheter and the associated short-term incontinence that occurs with the prostate's removal. The incontinence that can occur after the removal of the catheter occurs with either method. In this respect no advantage is gained with robotic removal. As previously discussed, when the prostate is removed, the male then depends on the external sphincter to regain continence regardless of the method chosen.

To highlight why the robotic removal is not an obvious choice for your prostate removal, consider again the laparoscopic removal of the gallbladder. In this case, there is a clear advantage of the laparoscopic method, which is most often performed as an outpatient procedure, with only a few small incisions, and requiring only a few days of recovery time, over the open method. In the case of the prostate, however, after laparoscopically (robotic) removal there is still the issue of needing to wear a catheter for a week or so and then the problem of incontinence after the catheter is removed. The time advantage that the laparoscopic method should offer is offset by the very nature of the surgery and the uncertainties of the effect of the prostate being gone. In my case, I had my prostate removed by the robotic method and did go home the next day, but I wore the catheter for six days, had hematuria (bloody urine) for weeks, and was totally incontinent for three months. I did return to work in about two weeks, but wearing a diaper. If you choose robotic over open, don't assume that the issues innate to removing the prostate will go away. In many ways the hype about the ease of seed therapy and the frequency with which patients choose this without a full knowledge of the effects of radiation on voiding are very similar to the hype related to patients choosing robotic surgery without knowing the specifics. The decision becomes less clear if you also consider that in some cases patients have to travel out of their home town for the surgery and that some robotic surgeons don't accept insurance. Below are the major factors regarding the two methods; you have to sort through what is important to you and be knowledgeable of the facts to make an informed decision.

> Oh, that the prostate was a gallbladder...
> Remove it and you'd be done.

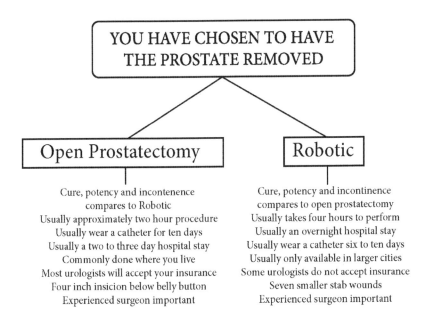

How I came to go the robotic route.

Once I decided to have the prostate removed, I did not look back. I remember being relieved that once I decided, it wasn't an issue that plagued me going forward. I felt fortunate that I was comfortable with it and had peace in my decision. It took me about three months to get there. What was surprising to me was how confident I was in my decision. I am not usually that way; I usually labor over the simplest of decisions. It is not uncommon for me to be in Wal-mart most weekends being "penny wise but dollar foolish," debating the cost of dog treats and fishing line. Because of the potential for the aforementioned risks, I did not want to have the procedure done in my hometown. I did not think it would be fair or appropriate to place the burden of a poor outcome on a colleague. I also did not like the idea of people that I work with daily in the operating room witnessing me having this particular procedure. Having my tonsils removed, a hernia repair, or something like knee surgery would have been different from what is involved with a prostatectomy. I mention these things to make the point that you too will have small, seemingly meaningless issues play an important role in your decision-making. Once I had decided on surgery, I then called the head guy at a respectable institution in Atlanta and queried him about the prospects of his performing an open prostatectomy. I might add that I never considered going out of Georgia for my procedure. Having done hundreds of the procedure that I needed, I felt there would not be a nickel's worth of difference in how someone did it here in Georgia as opposed to some major national referral center. Initially I did not favor, nor did I feel there was any advantage to the robotic method. I did not like the four hours of anesthesia (this, of course varies with the experience of the robotic surgeon) necessary to complete the procedure, and I basically felt more comfortable with the open method, as I was familiar with it. As it turned out, I did not get good vibes from the urologist I spoke to initially in Atlanta; he seemed more interested in touting his resume, and he repeated, an inordinate amount of times, how many of the procedures he had performed. He also stated that he left the catheter in for two weeks and that the procedure usually took him two and half hours to complete. That was about four days longer leaving in the catheter and about forty-five minutes longer to perform the procedure than I took. I did not get a good feel for the situation. Remember, a lot of this decision process is a gut feel. Around this time, a pharmaceutical representative came by our office and mentioned that he had had the robotic removal. (Remember how friends and family can factor in.) He was pleased with his particular doctor, but he had had an unusual bowel complication that complicated his course. Although he was pleased with the surgery, he stated that it took him about six months to get over the effects of the anesthesia and the bowel infection related to some antibiotics he received around the time of the surgery. (Remember the luck factor.) It is interesting to me that despite all the trouble he had after his surgery, I was not concerned that something untoward would happen to me nor did it influence my decision to have the prostate removed. I wrote it off to just, "stuff happens," and I think my experience as a surgeon helped me in not overly weighing an adverse event that happened to someone else. (Just because a friend does well or badly doesn't mean anything to you.) I called his surgeon and found him very down to earth. He did say he had done a lot of the robotic prostatectomies, which is what I wanted to hear, but the difference between his demeanor and the other surgeon's was dramatic. He really did not tout the robotic method as being much better in terms of cure and incontinence, which I knew to be true, but said, "I think I do a little better on the potency side." I liked him, and I liked what I thought was his realistic assessment of how the robotic method stacks up against the open method. I then began to think that I might get back to work a little faster with the robotic prostatectomy, and subsequently elected to go that route. I liked the fact that the hospital he used was just outside Atlanta and right off the highway and that I could get there the morning of my surgery. Some of what I experienced with my decision to have my prostate removed robotically was lucky and some was not. I still don't understand why it took me so long to be "diaper free." In any case, I used, in retrospect, almost all of the aspects of this book to come to my decision. The decision should be based on many factors that are given varying levels of importance by different patients. This decision is truly a journey and hopefully one with an optimal end destination.

You want radiation – *External beam alone, seeds alone, or combination therapy.*

I am guessing that if you have chosen radiation, you feel that the cure rates are similar to surgery and that if you are lucky, you can achieve a curative treatment of the cancer without all the hassle of having it removed. This desire (to have your cake and eat it too) is alright; just see it for what it is. (To thy own self be true.) If you are leaning toward radioactive seeds, you like the idea of an outpatient procedure, no incision, and a limited time wearing a catheter, usually just a day. You may favor seeds alone over external beam because you don't want to make the 42 trips to the hospital that this would require. You also believe that your underlying voiding symptoms are such that the effects of the radiation will be minor and certainly less than the risks that can happen with surgery. You are thinking you can get back to what you enjoy sooner and radiation will impact your job and family less. You have a friend or two who had radiation and they were pleased. I know what you are thinking, because I was thinking the same way. The time out from work required for surgery was huge to me. Once you have decided on radiation, the urologist will refer you to the radiation therapist, and he or she will ultimately decide upon the type of radiation that will be best for you. In general, if your Gleason's score is predominately 6 and the volume of disease is not too high, it may be that seed therapy alone is enough for you. If your parameters are less favorable (higher Gleason's score), and the biopsy suggests high volume disease or that your cancer is near the capsule (the outer aspect of the prostate similar to the rind of an orange), the radiation therapist may recommend the addition of external beam radiation as well. There are two schools of thought in this issue. One view is that seeds and external beam should be done together every time regardless of the results of the biopsy. The thinking is that if external beam is added to the radiation regimen, then the seeds can be placed in such a way as to spare the area around the urethra (attempting to limit the negative effects on voiding) and treat any cancer that may have gotten into the capsule, an area potentially not treated by using seeds alone. The other view is that you use the combination of seeds and external beam radiation only if the radiation therapist feels the biopsy and PSA parameters warrant it. Which of the two methods you use will be a collaboration between you and the radiation therapist. Of course, external beam alone is also a viable treatment option and is usually chosen by a non-surgical type patient (remember that seeds require anesthesia) and patients who do not mind the 42 trips to the hospital or radiation center to receive the treatment.

My trip to the radiation therapist –

> ## *No good deed goes unpunished – the radiation therapist was doing me a favor.*

My biopsy report was predominately Gleason's 6, and the volume was low. I felt I would be a good candidate for seed therapy. I especially liked the fact that I might have it done on a Friday, worn the catheter overnight, and then gone back to work on Monday. I called a radiation therapist I knew and told him about my recent diagnosis and biopsy specifics. Although I was not completely sure I wanted to pursue radiation, I did know that for me it was a viable option and that I needed to know if I was a suitable candidate for it. I decided to play out the initial evaluation with the radiation therapist and then, having the knowledge of his evaluation, I could better choose between the two methods. He told me that I would need to have my prostate mapped. I learned that this involved being catheterized (I have probably catheterized about a thousand people but had never had it done to me) and that an ultrasound would be performed to do the mapping to determine if my prostate was suitable for seeds. I went to the radiation department at the hospital one day at lunch, between seeing patients, to have this done. I undressed and got on the exam table and the radiation therapist and his female assistant attempted to place the catheter. They could not get it in, and all the attempts to "push it by" were very painful. I was thinking that this experience was good for me, maybe it would make me a better, more "sensitive" doctor. Being a urologist, I knew why the catheter would not go in. A median lobe of the prostate was probably the culprit, and the catheter was being blocked by this lobe. As unfortunate and uncomfortable as this situation was, it actually was helpful in my decision process. If I was already having some obstructive voiding symptoms, and if it was hard to place a catheter, then I might be someone who would have worsening voiding symptoms with radiation. (Every experience, good or bad, teaches you something, and you learn more from a bad experience than from a good one.) I suggested that they get a coude catheter, one familiar to urologists, which has a bend in it that allows the catheter to flip up and over the median lobe. I also suggested filling a syringe with lubricant and then injecting that into the urethra to further facilitate the passage of the catheter. (Urology tricks, it's all about the tricks, trust me.)

It now had been about 20 minutes of me on the table naked, with people looking me, scratching their heads over what to do, and waiting on the nurse who went to get the catheter I had suggested. The catheter arrives, the lubricant is inserted, and the catheter is placed into the bladder. The ultrasound is placed into the rectum and procedure is begun. I am getting a 101 class in being a real live patient, how it feels, and the humility it teaches. The prostate is mapped, resulting in a series of ultrasound pictures at various levels of the prostate. Of particular interest to the radiation therapist is the area at the anterior aspect of the prostate under the pubic bone, as well as the prostate's anatomy at its junction with the bladder. They got all the pictures to their satisfaction and proceeded to remove the catheter. It would not come out and the pulling required in attempting to remove it was again very painful. Urethral catheters have a balloon at the end that, when filled with water, keeps the catheter in the bladder so it won't slip out. Pulling on a catheter with an inflated balloon forces the balloon up against the bladder and prostate, and that was what was causing the discomfort. It was determined that the balloon had been mistakenly filled with the lubricant instead of water, and the balloon would not go down. So there we were, two doctors who were friends and who treat prostate cancer, albeit differently, along with nurses, looking at my private part with a catheter in that would not come out, all trying to figure out what to do. It now had been about 45 minutes, and it was time for me to be back at the office. We decided to irrigate the balloon repeatedly with water to see if we could flush out or dilute the lubricant and then let the balloon go down. We did this for about ten minutes and then, without warning, a pull on the catheter delivers the partially deflated balloon through my prostate and urethra. Did I mention that this all was very painful? I got dressed, we looked at the pictures, and there was some concern regarding how the prostate was positioned relative to my bladder. I was told, "We may need to do this again, but a catheter won't be needed." We decided to talk again after further review of the pictures and allowing time for me to recover from "being a patient." I went back to my office to see patients. When I voided, it felt like I was, as patients have told me, "peeing razor blades."

> You may feel that I am being critical, that I may be including this story to dissuade you from choosing radiation, but just the opposite is true.

First of all, I was grateful to the radiation therapist and his staff for seeing me during lunch and being honest about the pictures they got and the need for more. I know they must have been thinking, "No good deed goes unpunished," because they missed lunch also. For me, the trouble involved with placing the catheter helped me immensely in closing ground on my decision. Through this process I learned how important an individual's specific prostate anatomy and its relationship to the pubic bone and the bladder were to the adequate placement of the seeds and ultimate cure. It confirmed that I had an enlarged prostate and hence more risk for obstructive voiding symptoms after radiation. The process allowed me to ask meaningful questions of my radiotherapist colleagues, and they were very professional, helpful, and kind to me. What I would want for my patients, they wanted for me: a cancer, a treatment, and a patient that are appropriately matched. The fact that I labored over the decision and went to the trouble of having my prostate mapped for seeds is an indication of how hard the decision is to make. Oh, by the way, I passed on the radiotherapist's suggestion that we "take more pictures." I knew about all I wanted to know about my prostate at that point.

You want to do something else – *Just because it's new doesn't mean its better*

Another option is cryosurgery. This treatment is similar to brachytherapy in how it is performed and the need for anesthesia. Probes are placed into the prostate through the perineum, and the prostate is frozen. This procedure is usually performed by a urologist. The patient who chooses this option either doesn't want or for medical reasons cannot undergo surgery, has fears regarding radiation, or likes the fact that cryosurgery can be repeated if the PSA starts to rise at some point later in time. Cryosurgery can also be done after external beam radiation if it is felt that the cancer has reoccurred, and it is determined that the cancer is only in the prostate (i.e. there is no evidence of metastatic spread). Cryosurgery represents a small piece of the treatment pie in the USA, as the majority of patients elect to have surgery or radiation, and as such is not the focus of this book. I might add, if this book has helped you define your feelings between surgery and something else, it still has been very successful. Once you decide against surgery, then it is a matter of choosing between the other treatments. The first big decision is however, "is you for or is you against surgery."

Another, less likely option is HIFU (high intensity focused ultrasound), which is currently being performed in Canada, Mexico, and Europe but is not yet FDA approved in the United States. HIFU will probably be available in our country in upcoming years. It treats the prostate with ultrasound and is very similar to cryosurgery in terms of risks and benefits with some exceptions, most notably a better chance of preserving sexual function.

You want to do nothing - *Surveillance therapy is always an option.*

Primum non nocere - First do no harm.

Doing nothing is always an option, and, in fact, I give it as an option to every patient I see for any problem, particularly if "the treatment is worse than the disease." In regards to prostate cancer, doing nothing is referred to as surveillance therapy. Often a patient will quote something he read in the paper or heard about prostate cancer being slow-growing, and he questions the need for a biopsy. The specifics of the biopsy are the determining factor in the surveillance decision. You have to know you have prostate cancer first of all, and then you need to know the parameters of the biopsy to see if surveillance is a good option for you. In general, surveillance is considered if the patient is 70 or older, in marginal health, and the parameters of the biopsy are favorable. There is some risk that the cancer will progress; therefore the surveillance follow-up usually involves slightly more frequent rectal exams and PSAs. This is why this option is referred to as active surveillance. A decision to abandon the "do nothing" approach could occur when either the rectal exam or the PSA changes enough to warrant intervention. Physiologic age comes into play in the surveillance decision, because unless the biopsy parameters are very unfavorable (large amount of Gleason's 8 or higher), a life expectancy of less than five years would most probably result in demise from causes other than the prostate cancer. The literature is replete with studies on how patients fare after choosing surveillance, and for some patients, surveillance is the appropriate thing to do. Quality of life is an important factor in this decision.

An example is a 73-year-old patient with less than a five-year life expectancy and recently diagnosed with prostate cancer. If he has the "slow growing" type of prostate cancer and a relatively good quality of life, surveillance therapy is clearly the way to go. Surveillance gets a bit dicey if a younger patient, with many years at risk for progression of his cancer and unfavorable parameters in his biopsy, chooses this route. Some patients have heard that all prostate cancers are slow growing, so they make their decision to manage their cancer by surveillance therapy thinking the likelihood of progression is small. I have seen this scenario occur despite telling a patient that in his case, the unfavorable nature of his biopsy, his age, and his general health argued against this form of management. This shows how "a little knowledge can be a dangerous thing." Yes, surveillance therapy is a reasonable management option. Yes, most prostate cancers are slow growing. However, you cannot blindly mix the two concepts without considering the specifics to make your decision. Surveillance works best in the patient where the downside of the treatments outweighs the risks of the cancer. The patient who elects to take this approach is monitored by way of a rectal exam, serial PSAs and sometimes repeat biopsies to be sure there is not a change that would prompt treatment.

In my case, I considered surveillance, but because I had a small amount of Gleason's 7 (more aggressive grade) in my biopsy and a young age (increased years at risk), I felt compelled to do something to deal with the problem. It takes a certain type of mindset to pursue surveillance. The idea of an untreated cancer "in my body" loomed over me, and my "mentality" did not suit me for this approach. *Your* mindset may be different.

Representative case studies – *How other's decisions played out for them*

There are a myriad of potential outcomes if one considers all the variations of cure, potency, incontinence, and complications. Each of these elements varies as well in terms of their timeline and severity. The cases that follow are in no way exhaustive but do give a feel for what you might expect with a particular decision. All of the potential scenarios also show why you will get so many different opinions from the people you speak to about what and how they did with their prostate cancer decision.

Cases 1 and 2 are examples of surgical removal of the prostate that went well. Cases 3 and 4 are variations of surgical outcome. Case 5-8 are representative cases treated with radiation with varying results. All of the initials and biographies have been changed with the exception of J.M. (me). These case studies are generic in the sense that I have seen examples of each of these many times in my 20-year career. They are added to give you an idea of how there can be "variations on a theme" and, by doing so, aid you not only in making your decision but in allowing you to visualize how your decision could play out.

Case study 1: G.T.

Age 53
Physician-surgeon
Married with two young children
Health good, good underlying erectile function, no voiding issues
Pathology of biopsy: minimal volume/Gleason's 6/ both sides of prostate had cancer.

Bias toward surgery

Prostate exam: normal

Cure driven

Being a self-employed physician, time off from work was an issue, but trumped by desire for cure

Evaluated robotic removal but wanted to stay in local community. The desire to have people he knows working on him was very important to him and his wife.

Caveat: The fact that G.T.'s children were young and his years at risk were high weighed heavily in his decision to go for what he believed to be the most aggressive treatment, surgery.

Outcome: He had his prostate removed by the open technique locally in his hometown. (I performed the surgery.) He was in the hospital one day, wore the catheter ten days, his pathology demonstrated a Gleason 6, 5% of the prostate had cancer, and the disease was confined to the specimen. He was continent day one upon removing the catheter and is potent without medicines, but it took almost two years to achieve full erectile recovery. His PSA at two years is undetectable.

Case study 2: J.M.

Age 53

Physician

Married, three children all out of household (but not out of mind)

Health good, sexual function good, mild to moderate symptoms of obstruction

Pathology of biopsy: low volume/predominately Gleason's 6, both sides of prostate had cancer

Bias toward surgery

Prostate exam: normal

Cure driven

Self-employed and potential for missing work a major factor but trumped by need for cure.

Caveat: J.M. did not want to have surgery locally and was displeased with a surgeon at a large referral center in Atlanta who did open surgery. He gravitated to the robotic removal because of concerns regarding time out from work, and he liked the honesty of the robotic surgeon.

Evaluated seed therapy and had mapping of prostate by radiation therapist to determine suitability for seed therapy but elected not to pursue seeds. The initial thoughts regarding treatment were driven by work and expense of missing work, but over time cure and fear of radiation drove the decision.

Outcome: He had robotic removal of the prostate. One night in the hospital, wore a catheter for six days, wore a diaper/condom catheter for three months for total incontinence, pathology was low volume, Gleason's 6 and 7, cancer confined to the prostate. PSA at two and a half years is undetectable; he is now potent and continent.

Assessment

The above cases represent two very similar patients who both chose surgical removal, but by different methods and for different reasons. Both were lucky and have had a good outcome.

Case study 3: S.P.

Age 69
Retired
Married

Good health, marginal sexual function, significant obstructive voiding symptoms.

Pathology of biopsy: Gleason's score 6 and 7, moderate volume

Prostate exam: no nodule but two plus enlarged (B.P.H.)

This patient had no bias but was very aware of his obstructive voiding symptoms.

This patient's driving force in deciding to remove the prostate was his wife's and his desire for cure and being able to remove the obstructive voiding symptoms related to the enlarged prostate. Men who have had obstructive symptoms for years will sometimes develop hyperactive symptoms due to the bladder having to work harder to overcome the obstructive nature of the prostate. This in turn thickens the bladder wall musculature and causes what is called detrusor hyperactivity (irritative voiding symptoms, frequency, urgency, and nocturia). These symptoms are usually more prominent than the patient realizes as they come on slowly over the course of many years. The patient in this case had these symptoms prior to surgery, and it complicated his postoperative course. This patient did extremely well with the surgery and after two years is free of cancer, but continues to have incontinence from an urgency standpoint. He will have days that he is dry, and other days in which without warning his bladder will have a contraction and he will leak urine. Various medicines have been of limited help, and it has been a frustrating situation for the patient and his wife. He does not regret his decision, as he is pleased with a negligible PSA, but obviously the incontinence has hampered his quality of life.

Caveat: When urologists perform a TURP (transurethral resection of the prostate), prostate tissue is removed and results in opening the prostatic urethra. This improves obstructive voiding symptoms and is similar to taking "a core out of an apple" and often referred to by patients as having a "roto-rooter." Although obstructive symptoms will improve, any pre exisistent irritative symptoms will most probably continue, sometimes to the point of urgency incontinence.

What happens here is that with the restriction of flow corrected by the TURP, the urgency symptoms become more prominent. It can take weeks to months for the bladder to "calm down" and the urgency symptoms to improve. Sometimes they don't, particularly in older men whose symptoms have been present for a long time. It is my feeling that the surgical patient described in this case was experiencing this phenomenon. His situation would probably not be better if he had had radiation. If he had had radiation without doing something to relieve the obstruction before, his obstructive symptoms would have worsened, with no surgical options. If he had had a procedure to open the prostate before seeds, he would have still had the urgency symptoms from the detrusor hyperactivity in addition to the irritative symptoms related to the radiation. This case is just a difficult situation resulting from longstanding obstructive voiding symptoms that were more significant than the patient or the doctor realized preoperatively. This patient's current plight could not have been prevented, but a doctor can always do a better job of anticipating it and better prepare the patient and his wife for it.

Case study 4: S.P.

Age 65
Retired professor
Married
Good health, active, sexually active, mild voiding symptoms

Pathology of biopsy: bilateral disease, PSA 8

Bias toward surgery

Prostate exam: subtle irregularity

Discussion: This case highlights the problematic issue of stress incontinence that can be associated with surgical removal. This patient loves to hike, and although his surgery progressed well and his PSA has stayed negligible, he has continued to struggle with stress incontinence. If he hikes or works in the yard, he must wear a liner to protect himself. He has had an outpatient procedure to place bulking agents around the area of the bladder neck to add resistance and hopefully stop the incontinence, but this only marginally improved the leakage of urine. He is currently considering having a sphincter prosthesis placed to correct the problem surgically.

Caveat: Stress incontinence and the degree to which a patient may have it cannot be predicted, and as I have mentioned earlier, this is a big reason many patients do not choose surgery. It is also a luck issue. It happens commonly that procedures performed correctly and exactly the same way will result in a different outcome in different patients. It is something that is frustrating to both the patient and urologist.

Case study 5: J.R.

Age 63

Small business owner

Married

Good health, potent, active, mild obstructive voiding symptoms

Pathology of biopsy: moderate volume, mildly elevated PSA

Gleason's score predominately 6

Bias toward radiation

Prostate exam: normal

Cure important, but felt the percentages were about the same and, being self-employed, placed ease of treatment and time out from work at the forefront of his decision. He chose seed therapy followed by external beam radiation.

Caveat: J.R. is an intelligent patient who did massive amounts of research and made a decision that was well-thought-out and matched to his situation and needs.

Outcome: This patient had significant irritative and obstructive voiding symptoms for nine months. His radiation was performed with another team of physicians in a larger city elsewhere and he was referred to me because of the refractory and significant nature of his voiding problems. Numerous regimens of medicines were employed over several months to address his symptoms, which decreased over time. This was a very frustrating time for the patient because the urgent nature of his voiding associated with burning affected every part of his life. Part of this frustration was due to his complete surprise that radiation would cause voiding symptoms so severe and impact his life to such a degree. I developed a very close relationship with this patient, and after about a year of slowly retracting meds and the tincture of time, he improved. He now has a normal voiding pattern; he is on no medicines except for Viagra as needed. His PSA is normal. This patient also had a rise in his PSA at year two out from treatment. This rise is something common to brachytherapy and usually the PSA returns to negligible values with time. This bump in the PSA value and the symptoms related to voiding caused great anxiety in this patient and had not been adequately discussed with him pretreatment.

Assessment

This is a case of a patient making all the right decisions but having a very bumpy road after treatment with radiation that probably could not have been prevented. He may have had some mild to moderate underlying voiding symptoms that caused this scenario. He also had an unpredictable intense tissue response to the radiation. Several years out, he is doing well. This makes the point that if you choose radiation, you should maintain a good working relationship with the urologist. If you have voiding symptoms after radiation, it will be the urologist, not the radiation therapist, who will be working with you. This patient did not necessarily make the wrong decision; he just had the side effects of radiation, the severity of which cannot be predicted before treatment. This possibility should be in your personal database and used in consideration of your decision.

Case study 6: J.T.

Age 65

Company executive

Good health, good sexual function, no obstructive voiding symptoms.

Path report: 20% of the biopsies positive with Gleason's 6 and 7

Bias toward radiation

Prostate exam: subtle irregularity and PSA 6.8

This patient did not want surgery and felt radiation would be best for him. He was referred to a radiation therapist and, because of the rectal exam irregularity, had the combination of seeds and external beam radiation. Other than one month of mild/moderate irritative voiding symptoms, which gradually went away, he did quite well.

Case study 7: S.T.

Age 70

Retired

Fair health, sexual function marginal and not an issue, mild obstructive symptoms.

Path report: 50% of the biopsies positive and Gleason's 7

Bias toward radiation

Prostate exam: normal and PSA 6

This patient elected to have radioactive seeds. His age and medical condition made him a better candidate for radiation than surgery. Because he lived 30 minutes from the closest radiation facility, he elected to have seeds alone, thereby preventing the need for all the trips back and forth required by external beam radiation. Because of moderate obstructive prostate symptoms, cystoscopy was performed when it became apparent that he would choose seeds. This revealed an enlarged median lobe that was visually obstructing the prostatic urethra and was associated with changes in the bladder that indicated the patient was having more of an issue with voiding than he realized. (This is known as trabeculation, or enlargement of the muscles of the bladder indicative of obstructive voiding problems and is seen at the time of cystoscopy.) He underwent laser therapy to remove the obstruction, an outpatient procedure, and then had his seed therapy a month later. He had some irritative symptoms early on after the seeds, no obstructive symptoms, and most of his voiding symptoms improved over the course of one month. He had a good result in terms of symptoms, but it is too early to adequately evaluate the trending of his PSA, the ultimate determinant of whether any treatment of the prostate is successful. This case is a good example of using the method described in customizing a treatment plan to a patient's voiding situation, his "who are you" information, and his wishes regarding a decision. If you have elected to have seeds and you know you have obstructive voiding symptoms, it is imperative to deal with that issue *before* the seeds. You can surgically intervene for obstructive symptoms safely before seeds but operating after seeds can be problematic.

It better to cure at the beginning than at the end.

Case study 8: P.C.

Age 60
Coach
Good health, good sexual function, and no "subjective" obstructive voiding symptoms.
Path report: moderate volume and predominantly Gleason's 6
Bias toward radiation
Prostate exam: normal and PSA 7
Several things are interesting about this case. This patient had no *subjective* voiding symptoms at the time of his diagnosis of prostate cancer. The series of events which occurred following his radiation treatment and its dramatic affect on his prostate and prostatic urethra ultimately led to this patient experiencing longstanding difficulty voiding, irritative urinary symptoms and hematuria (blood in the urine). By subjective, I mean that when he was asked prior to treatment whether he had any voiding symptoms, he said no. He filled out a symptom score test, and this indicated no significant voiding symptoms. Despite his low symptom score and his feeling that he had no urinary problems; the urologist who performed cystoscopy (looking into the bladder and prostate with a lighted scope) after his radiation noted an enlarged

prostate and changes in the bladder consistent with bladder outlet obstruction. I have seen this phenomenon in men on many occasions in my career; the patient will tell you he voids fine, but all the tests indicate otherwise. These patients tell you there is no problem, and yet examination reveals excessive amounts of urine in the bladder even though the patient feels he has completely emptied his bladder. Often a patient's wife will have noticed that he spends longer in the bathroom or that she can hear the stop-start of urine flow. This situation occurs because the symptoms come on so slowly over time that the patient doesn't notice it. They will often comment that "sometimes two or three people do come and go in the restroom at restaurants before I can finish urinating." The importance of my pointing this out to you again, is to emphasize the need to assess your voiding pattern adequately prior to treatment, particularly if you are choosing radioactive seeds. This patient elected to have seeds and external beam therapy, and began experiencing difficulty voiding before the external beam portion was finished. Despite medicines, he labored to void for months, culminating in urinary retention and placement of a catheter. When given the option of either taking the catheter in and out to do voiding trials versus surgery to open the prostate, he chose the latter. His urologist performed a limited transurethral prostatic resection (the prostatic urethra is enlarged by trimming a portion of the prostate-similar to taking a core out of an apple) which improved his voiding pattern and made him catheter-free, but left him with irritative voiding symptoms and hematuria. I was asked to evaluate this patient several months later as a second opinion because of the persistence of blood and clots in his urine. When I examined the prostate with cystoscopy, the prostatic urethra was very angry in appearance and very little healing had occurred despite the time interval from the surgery. There was very little I could do for this patient other than reassure him that the prostate was open and that hopefully things would calm down and heal as time passed. This case represents a very difficult situation in which both the patient and the doctor had tough decisions to make.

Assessment

Several cases of radiation are presented, ranging from everything going well to a more complex scenario. The less than ideal instances don't take into account how the patients did in the long term with the cancer; they involve all the side effects. The focus of this book is here. I dare say that the last patient was probably very surprised to have had all the problems with urinating that he experienced. His case represents a situation gone awry and occurs uncommonly, but does occur. A lot of his problems related to bad luck, his body tissues being overly sensitive to radiation, and the fact that the full extent of his pretreatment obstructive voiding symptoms were not clinically apparent. There are similar cases in which urologists have been named in malpractice law suits for operating on a previously irradiated prostate. Because of this, urologists will be hesitant to perform operative procedures on patients who have had radiation for fear of the legal ramifications. (I can assure you that I personally will be very reluctant to do anything surgical on a previously irradiated prostate, not because it might not be clinically necessary or prudent, but for fear of a lawsuit if there is any untoward consequence of the procedure.) Had this patient had his obstructive symptoms dealt with prior to radiation, he probably would not have had all the obstructive problems after radiation. It is imperative to know if you have any obstructive voiding symptoms if you are planning to have seeds.

One of my favorite patients in my 20-year career was a retired girl's high school basketball coach. He had a state championship ring that attested both to his skills in coaching and the credentials to sponsor a summer basketball camp for girls at a local college each year in Gainesville, Georgia. I benefited from his camp in that he would bring me old t-shirts from the camp which I would in turn give to my children; they loved getting them, particularly my oldest son Clay, who loves basketball. He'd also bring me large cabbages from Clayton, Georgia; I loved seeing him coming because he was always bearing gifts. I was asked to see him for an elevated PSA, he was subsequently found to have prostate cancer, and he elected to have seed radiotherapy. He probably had more obstructive voiding symptoms than were known to him or me, and after the seeds were placed, he was unable to void. After several failed attempts to remove his catheter, he and I decided to place a supra pubic catheter (a tube that is placed through the abdomen just below the belly button directly into the bladder, thereby bypassing the prostate and the urethra) which he wore for about a year. I would run into Jack Griffeth, a radiation oncologist, from time to time and ask him when he thought it might be suitable for me to do something surgical to open the prostate and hence render this patient catheter free. I wanted to do something for this guy. I bet I asked him at least ten times over that period of time, "When can I do something?" Each time I asked he'd say, "If the patient will let you, it would be better to do nothing." I'd say, "It's been about a year now." He'd respond, "John, it's better to wait if he'll let you." Well this patient did let me. He never pushed me to do anything other than allowing the "tincture of time" to take effect. As I recall, he started dating someone with his supra pubic catheter still in; this amazing retired coach was in his early 70s at the time! We did voiding trials about every three months, and eventually he was able to void. He ended up getting married, again as I recall, around the time we were able to take the catheter out and leave it out. I remember this man as a beautiful, upbeat person who was obviously a positive mentor to thousands of young girls and despite adverse "urology issues" was able to begin a relationship that culminated in marriage and a honeymoon in Jamaica. My two boys and I still have his t-shirts as a memory to his spirit and love of coaching basketball. In retrospect, my radiation therapist was excellent counsel, and I'm glad I listened to him. This story also illustrates the role that the disposition of the patient plays in the management of an adverse medical situation. I think that if I were in his situation, I would have pushed my doctor to do something surgical in hopes of getting the catheter out, and then just cross my fingers hoping that "the art of getting away with it" protected me. A year is a long time to have a tube with urine in it coming out of your lower abdomen.

When urologists remove catheters for a voiding trial (to see if a patient can urinate), we commonly do it early in the morning. The thinking is that if there are any problems with voiding and a catheter needs to be reinserted, the urologist will be called during the day and not after hours at night. (Urology is often referred to as a "gentleman's" surgical specialty because there are few urologic emergencies at night.)

Urologic rule #1:
Don't buy shoes in the morning...
And don't pull tubes at night.

Part Five - The best-laid plans oft go astray

Medicine is an art, not a science.

Luck is when preparation meets opportunity. This holds true for the physician administering your treatment (doctors have good and bad days too) as well as for your ultimate outcome.

T he patient who has all the favorable parameters in terms of PSA and biopsy results, is appropriately treated by the urologist or radiation therapist, and makes the right decision for his specific circumstances can still have any or all of the aforementioned complications. This is why "the decision" is so important to make after careful consideration of all relevant factors. Neither a patient nor his physician can control luck, but a good decision can limit the untoward issues you can control. An example would be the patient with obvious obstructive voiding symptoms either choosing surgery or having a procedure before radiation to limit voiding issues after radiation. This patient has prevented one of the risks that he can control, and your decision should be tailored in the same way. The potential for unlucky and unexpected untoward events in the best of circumstances also explains why your physician usually will not push you to do a particular treatment even if he feels it might be best for you. In the case of a surgeon recommending surgery, this is somewhat of a protective maneuver on the doctor's part. If you do have one of the complications or risks, and you feel you were pushed toward surgery, you rightfully might blame the surgeon. You don't want that situation and the dirty little secret is that your doctors don't want it either. In my practice, the decision is clearly one that the patient makes with full knowledge of all the risks. You can, however, limit the untoward side effects by making the decision for the "right" reasons, and then hope you get a little luck on the side. All patients deal much better with issues as a result of any treatment when they have been informed and are aware of that possibility beforehand. I would not consider recommending surgery to a patient without having adequately educated him about the risks. A patient should thoroughly question his radiation therapist as to the potential side effects of various modes of radiation. This should include the immediate effect on how the patient will void and the long-term potential for negative influences on erections and tissues exposed to radiation.

The Luck Factor - *I'd rather be lucky than good, and I'd rather have good luck than have made the best decision.*

A surgeon is only as good as his last case.

> *God heals the patient; the surgeon renders the bill.*

*I have seen my surgeon only twice, once before the surgery and then during my hospital stay after the surgery. During the first meeting and after small talk and introductions, he asked me if I wanted to know any of the particulars of how he performed a robotic prostatectomy. I said, "No." He then asked, "Do you want me to do the lymph nodes?" I said, **"No, I just want to be lucky and for you to have a good day."** I added, "I do need directions to the hospital from interstate I-85."*

I had diagnosed a friend of mine with prostate cancer, and after several weeks of deliberation, he elected to have the prostate removed. He was at first troubled by whether to have radiation or surgery. I spent a couple of hours with him in the office as well as on the phone discussing surgical issues. He then spent over an hour in consultation with a radiation therapist, in addition to exhaustive personal research on his part. He interviewed several people he knew who had had both forms of therapy. He ultimately elected to have his prostate removed by the robotic method. A person could not have done a better job of vetting all the issues and researching treatments. On the day of his surgery, under anesthesia and after all the laparoscopic ports had been placed, the da Vinci robot malfunctioned. All of the instruments were removed; he was awakened and then placed in a holding area for six hours while the machine was fixed. He returned later that evening and again was put to sleep and the ports replaced. The surgery was then completed without incident on the second try. In this situation no one did anything wrong, my friend's decision was well thought out, and he just had some bad luck. I saw him walking in his neighborhood about three weeks after the surgery, and this is when he related to me the incident regarding the robot. He began to question his decision; why had he left his home town, what advantages did the robotic method give him, and were the two doses of anesthesia the reason that after three weeks he did not yet have his energy level back? Be prepared for a variation of this scenario happening to you regardless of the route you choose. "Medicine is an art not a science," and stuff happens.

Whether you elect to have radiation or surgery, how well you do depends a lot on just plain luck. The following truisms need to be understood regardless of how much time and effort you took in making your decision, which decision you made, or who you chose to treat your cancer:

- A radiation therapist cannot predict to what degree the radiation will affect your body, continence or erectile function. For reasons we do not know, different people and different prostates react differently to radiation with varying degrees of severity.

- A surgeon cannot tell you with certainty that you will be completely continent or potent after your surgery.

- Neither the surgeon nor the radiation therapist can predict whether or not you'll have a complication peculiar to the treatment chosen.

- A radiation therapist cannot tell you that you will be cured.

- A surgeon cannot tell you that you will be cured.

After radiation, you are lucky if:

- You have brachytherapy, and you have had placement of the seeds in such a way as to adequately treat and kill all the cancer in the prostate. The anatomy, or shape of the prostate, is different for each person, so that some prostates are easier to place the seeds in the most advantageous fashion. If you are lucky, the anatomy of your prostate lends itself to placement of the seeds.

• You have brachytherapy, the assessment of any underlying obstructive symptoms were fully vetted and dealt with before the procedure, and as a result you have no problems with voiding after the procedure.

• Your body responds to the radiation in such a way that you have little or no irritative voiding symptoms and, if they do occur, they persist for only a short time or are handled nicely by medications.

• Your baseline erectile function is such that the effect of the radiation on the nerves responsible for erections has minimal effect on your potency. If the radiation does hurt your erections, you're lucky if oral medicines correct it and you don't have some of the side effects related to the oral medicines.

• You have no long-term side effects related to the radiation.

• Your PSA reverts to a low point (hopefully a nadir of .5 or less) and stays there.

• You're cured.

After surgery, you are lucky if:

• The nerves are spared, and you are completely potent with or without the aid of medicines. The prostate's anatomy and how it is situated within the pelvis can affect the difficulty of the procedure and the ability to spare the nerves. Whether or not you have lucky anatomy won't be known until the surgeon does the procedure. (Just as the outside of peoples' bodies are different, so too is the anatomy on the inside. A narrow pelvis with lots of veins makes open removal very difficult. A prostate with a median lobe (a portion of the prostate that protrudes into the bladder) makes robotic removal much more difficult.

• You regain continence within a few weeks and have no or only occasional stress incontinence.

• You have no problems with the surgery in terms of anesthesia, infection, bleeding or other complications.

• The catheter doesn't bother you much, and you don't have bladder spasms.

• Your PSA stays undetectable for years after surgery, and no additional treatment such as radiation is necessary.

• You're cured.

• Upon reviewing the final pathology report, all the cancer was confined to the prostate with no seminal vesicle involvement, the Gleason score is predominantly 6, and the volume is low. If you have a small volume of disease but the location is at the seminal vesicles, then your chance of cure decreases.

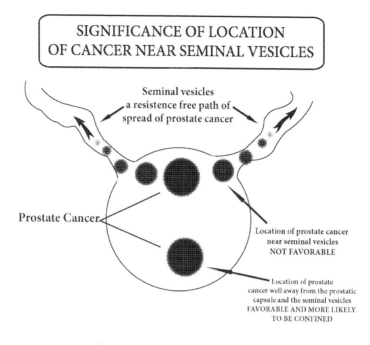

SIGNIFICANCE OF LOCATION
OF CANCER NEAR SEMINAL VESICLES

Seminal vesicles
a resistence free path of
spread of prostate cancer

Prostate Cancer

Location of prostate cancer
near seminal vesicles
NOT FAVORABLE

Location of prostate
cancer well away from the prostatic
capsule and the seminal vesicles
FAVORABLE AND MORE LIKELY
TO BE CONFINED

I mention bladder spasms above because of something that happened to me and because of experience with my patients whose prostate I have removed. The bladder is in essence a very large and strong muscle. Any manipulation of the bladder, including removing the prostate and then placing a catheter, can cause bladder spasms. A catheter is necessary after removing the prostate because you have separated the bladder from the urethra by removing the prostate, and the catheter allows for the drainage of urine while the new connection between the bladder and the urethra heals. This usually takes 7- 10 days, which is why you have the catheter in the length of time you do after surgery.(Please see the previous diagram of the prostate removed.) I have had several patients, one of whom was a friend of mine, tell me that the most painful part of the whole surgical experience was wearing the catheter and bladder spasms. This particular patient mentioned this fact to me at the time of his hospitalization and then asked me why I had not told him about it ahead of time. I told him it did not happen often, and, if it did, we had medicines, B and O suppositories in particular, to handle it. I remember listening to him discuss this issue, but I don't remember it making an impression on me to the extent that I began warning patients about it or taking other precautions to keep it from happening. A bladder spasm is very painful. If you have ever seen a professional football player collapse on the field because of a muscle spasm in his thigh, you then have noticed how they grimace in pain and have to leave the game. A bladder spasm is very similar to this, a very painful contraction of the bladder muscle that causes excruciating pain at the bottom of your abdomen. When I woke up in the recovery room after my prostate was removed, I experienced a bladder spasm first-hand, and it was the most horrible pain of my life. I am a wimp when it comes to pain related to dental work, but otherwise I am pretty good with pain. I have had three significant knee injuries with sports and subsequent surgery for each, so I know pain. Instead of waking up peacefully, feeling happy that my surgery was over and I was safe, I was in intense pain. I found myself having an ongoing dialogue with the recovery room nurse, who I believe was trying very hard to help me, about how badly I was hurting and the need for more pain medicine. She said, "You've already had 100 mg of Demerol." "Yes ma'am, but I am still hurting. May I have some more or something else? I may need a B and O suppository or maybe a couple of Levsin S.L.s, do ya'll have those?" After she put in the suppository to no benefit, she then brought me two sublingual Levsin S.L.s. The Levsin S.L. should dissolve immediately under your tongue and give almost immediate relief, but mine just sat under my tongue like little bricks and got stuck there, negating any benefit they might have had. I ended up having to chew them up into big chunks and then swallow them whole, just to get them out of my mouth. I continued hurting the entire time I was in the recovery room, and finally I told the nurse that the "100 mg" of Demerol she mentioned was "just a number" and that I needed more. I am sure that this remark came across as condescending, and she was probably thinking that I was just another one of those wimpy doctors who "can dish it out, but can't take it," and make bad patients; I may have been. After about 45 minutes of me hurting and asking for more pain medicine, in walked my doctor. "John, are you hurting?" "Yes, I think I am having a bladder spasm that will not break, and it is killing me. Is there something else you can do?" "What would you recommend, John?" Between groans I told him, "Well they've tried Demerol, Levsin S.L., and a B and O suppository, but nothing has touched this pain. How about giving me some morphine?" My surgeon looked at me somewhat puzzled as I writhed around clutching my lower abdomen and said, "Morphine, John? For a bladder spasm?" "I don't care what you give me, I'd like this pain to go away, please." **He said he'd order more pain medicine for me, and as he was leaving he said with a smile, "John, I had a good day."(This is exactly what I wanted to hear.)** *I said, "Thank you for what you have done for me." He ordered additional medication and the pain gradually went away about an hour after I returned to my room. My surgeon may not have appreciated the degree of pain I was experiencing. Despite my patients telling me for years how painful bladder spasms were, I did not fully "feel it" until I had one. My wife said she was fine throughout the whole process of my cancer journey until she saw me on the stretcher upon returning to the room, moaning with this bladder spasm. She said she had never seen me in that much pain. After the pain went away in the* *room, it never returned. Later my wife asked me if I thought I would be a better, more caring doctor now that I had been though this surgery and in particular this bladder spasm ordeal. I told her that as a rule I was fairly sensitive to patients' needs already and that my experience probably would not make much difference. About two weeks later and now sporting a condom catheter with a leg bag on underneath my scrubs, I am checking on a patient in the recovery room whose prostate I have just removed. I am wearing a condom catheter because the amount of urine I was leaking filled a diaper in less than an hour, and a prostatectomy usually lasts two. As irony would have it, the patient is having a bladder spasm, and as I arrive he is clutching his lower abdomen and pleading with the nurse to give him medicine for the pain. "He has had 100 mg of Demerol," the nurse says as I approach. He tells me this while indicating by his facial expression that he thinks the patient either has a low pain tolerance or is just pretending to be in pain to get more pain medicine. I saw myself lying there. "I am not as interested in the number of milligrams of medicine he has had; that is just a number. I am more interested in the relief of his pain; please give him more until his pain is gone." I stayed in the recovery room, and he got more medicine until he was comfortable. The point of the above story is two-fold. For one, I am a more sensitive doctor having had this surgery and all the things that went with it, from being told the biopsy had cancer to dealing with the surgical aftermath. More importantly for this section of the book, I am making a point about luck. Don't forget the role the luck factor plays in how well a decision pans out. There is no way to predict if a surgical patient will have bladder spasms or, for that matter, any other potential complication. I was unlucky in that regard and for no reason. A well thought-out decision, qualified doctors, and a little luck are what I am hoping for for you. At every step of your treatment, no matter what you decide to do, there is an opportunity for your situation to go well or not. There are issues about your anatomy, your cancer, your doctors, and how your body responds to treatment that cannot be predicted. You need to know this and be aware and prepared for the possibility of things not going precisely as planned.*

A "trifecta" (Cured, continent, and potent) is what you want, but might not be what you get.
And that is why-
Medicine is an art, not a science.

Epilogue - Now that you know, tell others

> *Shared joy - twice joy – Shared sorrow - half sorrow*

I t goes without saying that an important and vital aspect of your journey is to share your situation with friends and loved ones. As we have discussed, their input will be important in helping you make your decision. The focus of what I want to discuss with you now, however, is how you choose to help others now that you are an expert and have "been there, done that." What most patients tell others who have been newly diagnosed depends a lot on how they did with the treatment they chose.

Patients who do well and have a good result tend to take ownership and pride in their decision, the method of treatment they chose, and the doctor who did it. In this case, when this patient learns of a friend who has been recently diagnosed, he will usually search him out and most likely advise him to do what he did. I'm not sure from where this particular attitude originates; it is almost as if having had a good result by a certain physician reflects well on the patient's decision making. Imagine in your mind's eye, the patient with a puffed up chest saying to the newly diagnosed patient, "I chose to do this, and I used so and so, and he was wonderful. I am doing great." I, as the physician, have benefited from this type of "advertising" and am very much aware of the need to "re-educate" the new patient of all the pitfalls of the various treatments. I make it clear that if another patient did well with surgery, it doesn't mean that he will or that it is the best and most appropriate method for him. This is analogous to the chance of flipping a coin and getting heads three times in a row. The odds of getting three heads in row are very low, but the odds of a head on the last flip are the same as each of the other flips: 50-50. In other words, you will have the same initial risk as your friend; the fact he did well does not improve the chances that you will. All the potential risks begin anew when it is you undergoing the procedure, regardless of who is doing the procedure or how your friend did.

In the opposite situation, you have the patient who chooses a well-thought-out treatment plan and has a bad result. This patient is often hard on himself for making a decision that resulted in having a particular complication and begins to wish he'd done something different. "I'd have never done it this way if I had known this was going to happen," is something I hear often. I do believe I hear this more often from patients who elected to have radiation than from those who have had surgery. I am not being critical of radiation; I believe this is because patients understand the risks associated with surgery, but don't fully comprehend how radiation affects voiding, sexual function, or the potential for issues down the road. Unhappy patients tell others not to do what they have done. There is a saying that "a happy patient will tell 20 people, an unhappy patient will tell a hundred." The unhappy situation and the patient's retelling of it do not tell the whole story either, and this is not fair to the treating physician or helpful to the newly diagnosed patient. The bad result is reported without attention to all of the other issues previously discussed, and, of course, don't forget the luck factor.

So how should you help others? First of all, become an advocate for early detection. Tell your friends to be sure to have a rectal exam with a PSA each year starting around age 40. Some may tell you that 40 is too young. It is uncommon to have prostate cancer at that age, but it does happen. There is also a benefit to having a history of PSA trends over time, which will help the urologist in evaluating the need for a biopsy. The increase in my PSA over time is what prompted me to have a biopsy. If you want to share your experiences with the treatment you chose with a newly diagnosed patient, feel free to tell him your story, but for the reasons I have delineated, don't advise them on what to do. Explain that the options are complicated and the risks varied, and that what was best for you may not be the best for them. Encourage them to work through the "who are you" scenarios, the specifics of their disease, and seek the counsel of their physician.

> Your story becomes part of their database of what they *could* do, not the template for what they *should* do.

Determining who you are, what is important to you, and where you are in life, as well the specifics of your cancer, all play a role in arriving at *your* decision. Use your family physician, urologist, or radiation therapist to help sort through all you have gleaned from research, friends, family, and your own soul searching. Ultimately the decision will be a culmination of your assessment of this knowledge in the context of what is important to you and your particular situation. In time, as I did, you'll arrive at a decision that just feels right for you, a "gut feeling" so to speak. Then just go with it, don't look back, and hopefully the stars will be aligned for you. I hope that my journey, told through an eclectic mix of medical and personal experience, stories, and humor, will be of help to you in your journey to "the decision."

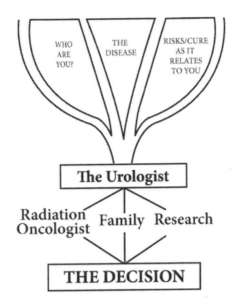

You may feel that I am assigning a more prominent role in the "decision" to the urologist than is justified or fair. However, your urologist is the one that did your prostate biopsy and told you that you have prostate cancer. Your urologist was the first caregiver to speak to you about your disease and discuss the treatment options with you and your family.

> *For better or worse, the urologist is the prism through which your decision must pass.*

What the above illustration shows is that your ultimate decision is multi-dimensional; it all starts with a urologist but it ends with you using everything "in your quiver" and everybody at your disposal to make a decision that is right for you.

Extras – Always give 'em a little more than they paid for

*W*hen my children were young I purchased several hundred dollars' worth of magic tricks in which the success of the trick was based more on its cost than my skill as a magician. The more I spent on the trick, the easier it was to perform and the more it appeared as magic. I had about 30 of them, and my favorite was a handkerchief that had a bra hidden inside. To perform the trick you ask a woman, usually the teacher of my particular child at the time, to place the middle part of the handkerchief into the front of her blouse or shirt. I would place a student on each side of the teacher with each holding an end of the handkerchief. After saying "abra cadabra," I would instruct them to pull each end. This resulted in the middle part popping out as a bra. I would very quickly gather up the bra and handkerchief and exclaim, "Oh my goodness, I am so sorry." It was a big hit every time I did it, and of course the trick cost a lot. On one occasion after I'd performed the trick for my son Sam's second grade class, a grandmother of one of the students approached me at a P.T.A. function: "John, my grandson told me something very interesting this afternoon. He said, 'Grandma, you should have been in my class today. Dr. McHugh did a trick and took Ms. Wolfe's panties off!'"

Something else interesting occurred after the bra trick in Ms. Wolfe's classroom that day. As I was gathering up my magic tricks, she approached me and whispered into my ear," John, what makes that trick so remarkable is that I haven't worn a bra since the seventies."

A patient of mine who had prostate cancer and whose prostate I had removed told me one day during a visit that he was a clown, but he could not do tricks. I told him about my little show, and over the next few years I did several "events" with him where he'd do the clowning and I'd do the tricks. As a gift he gave me an excellent clown book on making balloon animals. Before each example of an animal there would be a saying; I remember two distinctly. The first: Don't show up to a performance with alcohol on your breath. The second: Always give 'em a little more than they paid for. Both sayings have served me well over the years as a surgeon. My clown friend passed away several years later due to lung disease that resulted from his inhaling cement dust during a mission trip. He died with a clown figurine dangling from the ceiling above his bed in his hospital room. So, here you go, what follows is "a little more than you paid for," in honor of a clown who was both a patient and a friend.

Patients do the funniest things.

Curious things that patients have done or said to me when the subject of prostate cancer came up or the diagnosis of prostate cancer has been made known to them. Do you see yourself in any of these examples?

The following examples represent the meshing of the two sayings, "clever by half," and "a little knowledge is a dangerous thing." In a lot of these incidences, you'll see that the patient has a bias that he can do the research on his own and make a decision on that alone. You will also see a trend in patients who behave this way to hold the bias that the surgeon himself has a bias, toward surgery, i.e. "Why even discuss it with him, I know what he'll recommend."

- Fly from Georgia to somewhere in the Northeast to have a community urologist surgically remove the prostate, in the same way I would have performed the procedure here, and then return to me to remove the staples and ask me to manage a wound infection as a result of the surgery. This patient had a friend who had had his surgery there and had done well, and this was the basis of his decision. No inquiry to me for my advice.

- Drive 17 hours round trip twice, once for the office visit and once for the robotic surgery, because this patient's internet research indicated that a particular doctor in Louisiana was the best. At the time, Atlanta, less than one hour away, had two qualified robotic surgeons. I was not consulted.

- Despite high volume and high Gleason score on the biopsy, a patient declines treatment because he read that people "die of it, not with it," and he did not want "air to touch it." This patient was in good health and in his 60s.

- A patient declines a biopsy of the prostate, despite a PSA of 18 (normal is 4), because he read that having a biopsy was painful, and a friend had confirmed this. Despite explaining to the patient that we could use pre-biopsy pain medicines and I.V. sedation, he would not change his mind.

- Electing to be treated by radiation or surgery purely "because my brother had it done that way, and he did great."

- Electing to use herbs recommended on the internet and obtained from Mexico.

• Flying to a respectable institution somewhere up north on several occasions so he could be in a "study" for surveillance therapy. No treatment was done; he is just flying back and forth for blood work.

• Having cryosurgery done without any questions to me about my opinion regarding that procedure, and then returning to me for follow up. This patient was surprised that he was impotent, despite medical literature stating that this form of therapy has the highest impotency rates. When I informed him of this, he said, "My friend said it had the best rate of sparing potency." This is a good example of a patient "going it alone" and assuming that a urologist will always recommend surgery, and therefore not asking his opinion, and placing too much credence on what he had read or heard from friends.

• A patient who is on home oxygen, to whom I recommend external beam radiation because of his lung disease, insists that he wants robotic surgery. A friend of his at church had had robotic removal. Despite my mentioning that robotic surgery required usually four hours of anesthesia with great risk to him, he is planning to see a robotic surgeon for a second opinion. This is a very good example of "what may be best for the cancer is not best for the patient," and the importance of understanding the concept of years at risk for dying of prostate cancer. In this patient, who had favorable biopsy parameters and a medical condition that will certainly affect his longevity; a treatment that is less aggressive and without operative risks is best suited for him.

• (After informing a patient and his daughter that the prostate biopsy showed prostate cancer), the patient quickly says, "You can just put up your knife cause ain't nobody gonna cut on me!" At that point and time, there was nothing I could say or do to convince this patient otherwise that "cutting on him" may or may not be the most appropriate treatment for his prostate cancer.

• Choosing radiation because a commercial on the radio said that it would "cure" prostate cancer.

• Showing me a colorful brochure that he got in the mail and telling me, "I want my records, I'm going here." No questions to me about my opinion.

• (After having performed a rectal exam on a patient and informing him that it was normal), he asked if that was all I was going to do to check the prostate. I responded that a blood test, the PSA, would be done as well, and if it were normal, that he'd be good for one year in terms of checking on the prostate. He said that he wanted the digital test he had read about on the internet. I explained that we sometimes use the ultrasound to guide prostate biopsies, but that I was not aware of technology for a digital test of the prostate. (After insisting that he had read that a digital test was always done and implying that I might be behind on urologic technology), I determined that he was actually referring to a digital exam of the prostate, in other words, a rectal exam done with a gloved finger, or digit, which I had just performed.

• A patient and friend who was 49 asked me at a party when he should have his prostate checked. I said that the blood work and exam could be done in less than five minutes. I told him he could come by anytime at the end of his work-day through my office's back door, and I'd do the exam for free. He said that he was having no symptoms. I said that having no symptoms is irrelevant. He then told me he had had a colonoscopy and asked if that checked the prostate. I said no, that was a different organ. He said, like most people, "Isn't prostate cancer a disease of old men?" I said, "No," and mentioned that Frank Zappa died in his 50s, three years after the diagnosis of prostate cancer, adding, "It can be a painful death.", I said making the point that it would be prudent for him, at age 49, to be checked. My friend then said, "But Frank Zappa had a bad lifestyle." I replied that lifestyle was irrelevant as a risk factor for prostate cancer. In the matter of a two-minute conversation with this college-educated friend, he had verbalized almost all the half-truths regarding prostate cancer. He confirmed to me yet again why prostate cancer is often times diagnosed late, and revealed to me another damaging half-truth I'd never heard before: the "But I don't have a bad lifestyle" objection to having a rectal exam.

The question about, if a colonoscopy checks the prostate, comes up often. The answer is that, no, a colonoscopy does not check the prostate. The rectal mucosa drapes itself over the posterior aspect of the prostate, so, that when the gastroenterologist performs a colonoscopy, the prostate is not examined, as only the mucosa of the rectum and colon is seen.

The above explanation answers another common question; how is the tissue from a prostate biopsy is obtained? This is a good question. When a urologist performs a ultrasound guided prostate biopsy, the needle goes through the rectal mucosa into the prostate to obtain the necessary specimens. In the majority of instances there is no consequence of the procedure. Three percent of the time, however, an infection is caused by the prostate biopsy needle carrying bacteria from the rectum into the prostate. The rectal mucosa, the majority of the time, is very forgiving of the twelve to sixteen puncture wounds required of the procedure.

• On one occasion I went into an exam room that was "standing room only" to inform the patient and his extended family the results of the prostate biopsy. The family was sitting around the fatherly-looking man situated at the center of the group, as if he were the king, in a chair. As I sat on the exam table and look up from the pathology report, I slowly and deliberately say, "Mr. Smith, I have the results of the biopsy, and it shows a small amount of prostate cancer." The room was very quiet, as all of his family's eyes were lovingly and discernibly then directed to Mr. Smith to gauge his reaction. He then lets out a large and very audible sigh. He says, "Thank goodness! I have been paying on that cancer policy for 20 years, and it's about time I got to use it."

•At the time of a prostate biopsy a patient informs that he had had one of the first robotic surgeries performed in Georgia to replace the mitral valve of a heart. He then added empathically," If I have to have my prostate removed, I want it done with the robot!" This patient had had a good result using the robot (a machine mind you) by a doctor of a different specialty, on a different organ and with diametrically different post operative issues. However, he was transferring his previous unrelated positive experience to the treatment of prostate cancer. This breaks so many rules: the one dimensional decision maker, apples to apples, little knowledge, and the "go it alone" patient. You are right there with your doctor, ask him or her all the questions and get their opinion. And another thing, when it comes to having surgery, you don't ever want to be "the first one."

• The farmer from the mountains in overalls with limited ability to read and write simply saying to me: "You tell me what to do, and that is what I'll do." As simplistic as this seems, if you have the right doctor, it is a very smart approach to reaching your decision.

• Here's one on me…

After learning of my diagnosis, I began to read extensively about causes of false-positive readings on prostate biopsies hoping one might apply to my biopsy. (False positive means that the report says cancer, but in actuality there is no cancer.) I knew that with the quality of our local pathologists and the frequency with which they evaluated biopsies for prostate cancer, an error on their part would be most unusual. Just like you now, I began looking for a way out of this "major inconvenience." I was guilty of not simply consulting the pathologist, just as I have been critical of patients not consulting me. I found an article about using certain stains to confirm that there is not an error in the reading, called the pathologist, and asked him to perform these stains in hope that this prostate cancer thing was just a "misunderstanding." I asked him to do this; I did not ask his opinion or whether he thought it would be worthwhile. The pathologist consented and said that he'd get back to me with the results in a couple of days. A few days later (by the way, all the stress of waiting on the biopsy report happened to me all over again), I received a call. "John, this is Mark, the stains confirmed prostate cancer." "Thank you," I said, my hopes extinguished. "One other thing John, the stains revealed an additional area of cancer on the other side of the prostate, and it is Gleason's 7." A week later I got the $2000.00 bill from a pathology lab for all the special stains I had requested for the second reading. The "clever by half" syndrome that has plagued *me with so many things hit me yet again. When I advise you not to do certain things, I know of what I speak on many levels.*

Did you know?

• You have a higher incidence of bladder or rectal cancer after having received radiation.

• Frank Zappa, Bill Bixby, and Dan Fogelberg died in their fifties from prostate cancer, all within three years of diagnosis.

• One in six men will be diagnosed with prostate cancer at some point in his lifetime.

• Prostate cancer is the most common cancer in men.

• The reason the urologist will monitor the PSA after treatment with either form of therapy is that a PSA elevation over time is an indicator of recurrence of disease.

• The PSA is sometimes unreliable in the diagnosis of prostate cancer, but it is an excellent marker in determining the recurrence of prostate cancer after treatment.

• Prostate cancer is hereditary, so if your father has it, you need to be checked earlier and more often.

• Annually, 40,000 women die of breast cancer; 25,000 men die of prostate cancer. Government funding for breast cancer is twice that for prostate cancer.

• Prostate cancer is more common in African Americans and has a higher incidence of being more aggressive.

• The ribbon for breast cancer is pink; the ribbon for prostate cancer is blue.

• September is prostate cancer awareness month and designated as such in 2003 by President George Bush.

• October is breast cancer awareness month and designated as such in 1985.

• After the child bearing years the prostate has no other function than contributing to the fluid expressed at ejaculation.

• When a man has a vasectomy or a prostatectomy his sex drive or libido, which is dependent on the male hormone testosterone, does not change. Testosterone is produced by the testicles and released into the blood stream and subsequently not affected, or its blood level diminished, by either procedure.

One of the oldest Urology jokes around involves a man coming to the Urology clinic for a vasectomy all dressed up in a tuxedo. When asked," Why the formal attire?" he responds," If I am going to be impotent, I'm going to look impotent." The problem with this joke, as explained in the bullet above, is that a vasectomy makes you sterile (no sperm), it has no affect on potency. Potency refers to erectile function which is independent of fertility (which is what a vasectomy affects). I mention this because it is misconceptions like these which abound within the male population, and contribute to the "perfect storm" of delayed diagnosis alluded to earlier in this book.

• The external sphincter, which is anatomically below the prostate, is not disturbed by the prostate's removal. The contraction of this muscle contributes to the feeling of climax and is usually not affected by a prostatectomy.

At a three month follow up visit, with a patient in whom I had removed his prostate, I asked if he had had sexual activity. He indicated that everything was working well but that his wife would no longer have sex with him. "When I climax now doc, I start to shuttering all over so bad that it scares my wife. She won't have sex with me now, she's afraid I'm going to hurt something."

• After a prostatectomy the male and female anatomy, from a urinary standpoint, becomes very similar, except for the length of the urethra.

• The normal prostate is the size of a walnut, but can increase with age to the size of a lemon or sometimes larger.

• Men are often told they have an "enlarged prostate" after a rectal exam by their primary care physician. What is felt on exam does not give an indication of the prostate's anatomy as it pertains to the prostatic urethra. This is why a small prostate can produce significant obstructive voiding symptoms and a palpably enlarged prostate can cause no voiding symptoms.

• You can have prostate cancer without any voiding symptoms. You can have significant voiding symptoms and not have prostate cancer.

• You can have a very small prostate and have cancer or a very large one without prostate cancer.

• You can have an elevated PSA and not have prostate cancer. You can have a normal PSA and have prostate cancer.

• You can have a normal rectal exam and have prostate cancer. You can have an abnormal rectal exam and not have cancer.

• You can have the free portion of the PSA be very high, indicating a less than 5 percent chance of having prostate cancer, and a biopsy report subsequently showing every one of the twelve cores containing cancer.

• I perform several hundred biopsies a year and in approximately 15 percent of the men tested the biopsy reveals prostate cancer. Nationally the positive biopsy rate is probably somewhere between 15 and 20 percent.

• The most common reason for a prostate biopsy being done is for an elevated PSA.

• There are no hard and fast rules short of a prostate biopsy in determining if a man has prostate cancer. The pre-diagnosis variables are all over the board. (As residents) we used the term "mental masturbation" to describe when the options regarding a diagnosis or treatment were overly "cogititated" to the point of inaction (similar to a general who is indecisive to a fault). When there are any concerns that a man might have prostate cancer, in my opinion it is best to do the biopsy and put the issue to rest; it takes about 10 minutes to do, can be done in the office, and has a low risk profile.

• A rectal exam does not cause the PSA to be elevated.

• Having sexual intercourse the night before the PSA is drawn does raise the PSA.

In completing a medical questionnaire, a doctor asks an elderly lady," Do you and your husband have intercourse?" The lady goes to the waiting room door and yells in front of all the waiting patients and asks, "Honey do we have intercourse?" The husband, obviously perturbed by the question, says, "How many times do I have to tell you? We have Blue Cross Blue Shield!"

• If you have voiding symptoms because of prostate cancer, it is most likely in an advanced stage.

• The prostate, on rectal exam, feels like the thenar eminence, the muscular area on the palm of the hand below the thumb, when the fist is clinched.

• Prostate cancer is the single most common form of solid tumor in humans.

• Prostate cancer is second only to lung cancer in annual cancer deaths of U.S. men.

• I would rather have my prostate removed by a skilled open surgeon than an unskilled robotic surgeon, and vice versa.

• It is not uncommon for men whose prostate has been removed to have the loss of urine at the time of climax. This usually occurs if the bladder is relatively full and improves as the external sphincter matures in its new and heightened role in preventing incontinence.

• Urine is sterile.

• Surgeons are more afraid of veins than arteries. The anatomic variation of the veins surrounding the prostate can be a major cause of blood loss during a radical prostatectomy. Arteries are seldom an issue.

It invariably happens that after performing a rectal exam, a patient will ask, "So, tell me doc, what made you decide to go into this field?" What they are really asking is, "Why in the world would someone voluntarily choose to do this type of work everyday? All those years of study just to be a prostate doctor doing rectal exams on men all day?" The reason I went into urology is because it is one of the few surgical specialties that has limited exposure to emergencies after hours. Around the time that I had to declare what type of doctor I wanted to be, we had our first son Clay, and I hated spending nights away at the hospital. Someone told me that the urology program's residents took call from home, something none of the other surgical programs allowed. When I learned this, I immediately inquired, "Where do I sign up?"
When I called my mother to tell her I had decided to be a urologist, she exclaimed incredulously," Ye Gods John! Do you know what they do?"

The company that makes the da Vinci robot has become very successful, not only in terms of profitability, but as well, by facilitating its purchase and use in second tier sized communities across the U.S. My community of Gainesville, Georgia, a town of about 40,000, recently acquired one. That the marketing campaign has been so pervasive and successful reminds me of something I found hand written in one of my grandmother's books from the State Normal School in Athens, Georgia circa 1910.

He that burns the midnight oil
Will earn his way to fame…
He that sells the midnight oil
Will get there just the same.

Prostate Stories -
*Only a urologist
could write a story
in which the main
character is a
prostate.*

The Diaper Diaries - A screenplay

Scene one

In a garage a husband and wife are talking while cats are swirling about on top of a truck hood where they are accustomed to being fed, and they are each scooping out cat food with noses upturned.
"So when are you going to do something?" the wife asks.
"I don't know," the husband answers.
"What are you going to do?" the wife asks.
"I don't know," the husband answers.
After a kiss to the husband's cheek and the cats having been fed, the wife goes one way into the house and the husband the other way into his van.

Scene two

In the van, music blaring inside, and outside the window of the van the landscape is whizzing by. The husband, John, is tapping his hands on the steering wheel to the song and is singing along.
"One, two, three, four." *The upbeat start of the song.*
He talks to himself.
"The only reason they are playing this version of 'St. Peppers Lonely Hearts Club Band' is to set up 'A Day in the Life' I guarantee it."
He sings the remainder of the song and then waits to confirm that the radio station continues with 'A Day in the Life,' which the radio station does without an interruption. He is singing along in the car and the movements of his upper body and hands are

exaggerated and done as if conducting an orchestra. (He may or may not be eating cereal from a large bowl while driving, intermixing the eating, with the singing, with the turning of the steering wheel and playing drums.)

He points out to himself the alarm going off in the song and turns up the volume to accentuate it, and then says, "I bet they won't let us hear the piano for 45 seconds at the end."

He turns into a parking space behind an office. A commercial interrupts the piano sound at the end of the song. "I knew they'd do that." *he says as he gets out of the car and walks quickly toward the back door of the building.*

Scene three

The camera is moving and following John out of his van, into the office door, into the bathroom to swish his mouth with mouthwash and then put on a lab jacket. He goes to an exam room door, takes a chart off the door and begins to look at it.

Non-descript music is wafting down from speakers in the ceiling above his head.

A nurse appears, adjusts the collar of his jacket and says,

"Dr. Turner returned your call, you have patients in rooms 9 through 12, there is a specimen for you to look at in the lab, and Jenny and Johnna said they would be here at ten to talk about the party."

He walks into the room and begins looking at the chart as he sits on a rolling stool. There are a man and woman waiting and both have looks of concern.

John says, "Good morning, I'm sorry I am late, but I have good news for you, the reports show that the cancer has not spread anywhere and appears to be only in your prostate."

The couple sighs in relief.

John asks, "Have you decided what you are going to do?"

The man quickly answers, "Yes, I want to have surgery to remove it, and I want you to do it."

John glances at the time.

"I would like to speak to you in more detail about the surgery, but I need to attend to something for a few minutes... Will you please excuse me?"

Scene four

John is at a cluttered desk on the phone.

"Dr. Turner, my name is John McHugh. I am a urologist in Gainesville, I recently found out that I have prostate cancer, and I was wondering if you would agree to remove my prostate."

Scene five

John is walking to a small conference room where two ladies are waiting; they are wearing scrub suits and obviously work in the medical profession.

John says, "How are the plans for our party coming along?"

One of the ladies says, "Great, we've ordered the porta-potties, Dr. Francis's son is going to DJ, the barbeque will be catered by Johnny's, and we bought 25 cases of beer; everybody in the operating room is getting really excited. I bet there will be over 100 people from the operating room staff coming."

John says, "Everything alright with the money?"

The other lady says, "Yes. We just need a check for the beer."

John says "O.K., I'll have Keith give you a check; is he still planning to have a Corona bar with limes?"

The first lady says "It's all set up; he has gotten inflatable palm trees and tiki stuff at Wal-mart. Can we go out to your lake place the night before to set some stuff up?"

John says "Sure." He pauses. "There is something I need to mention to you."

John's nurse interrupts: "You have people waiting in rooms 10 through 12"

He looks at the nurse and says, "Thank you," then continues with the ladies.

John has piqued their interest and concern, and it shows on their faces and demeanor.

"There is a small chance I may not make it to the party."

With faces of shock the ladies say in unison "What?"

John says, "I'll tell you more later, but I have a medical issue I am dealing with, and it may affect my attending. I'll let ya'll know more later. Just keep up the good work and bring this thing together."

John stands, shakes hands, says "Thanks for all y'all have done," and then leaves.

The ladies stay seated and look at each other in puzzlement.

John returns to the clinic area to see patients again. As he pauses at the exam room door he hears the Beatles' song 'The End', motions to his nurse to come over to him nearer the ceiling speaker, and says "Watch this." John then plays the drum solo on his chest with his hands perfectly in pace with Ringo doing a drum solo. He says "How about that!" The nurse shakes her head; John enters the room with "Good morning, I'm sorry I'm late."

Scene six

John is back in the room with the first patient and has a chart explaining the anatomy of the prostate, how the anatomy looks with the prostate out, and why removal of the prostate causes leakage of urine. He is drawing the before-and-after picture on the paper covering of the exam table as the patient and his wife look on. Another song is drifting down from the ceiling in the background.

John says, "The only difference in the male and female anatomy in terms of how you urinate is the prostate. When the prostate is removed, the male anatomy in this regard becomes very similar to a woman's, which is why men will leak urine for a while after this surgery."

John draws a simplistic picture of a bladder, prostate, and urethra, and then after drawing lines to show where the prostate is removed, he draws another picture of just the bladder and the urethra.

John says, "After the surgery and once the catheter is out, you'll want to get some diapers. You'll need them for a few weeks."

The wife is more interested in this than her husband and moves forward to ask,

"Any particular kind? Did you mean diapers or a protective pad?"

John flippantly says, almost as a brush off, "It doesn't matter, whatever they have at a grocery store; I would think a diaper is a diaper. That may be the least of his worries."

Scene seven

John is in a hospital bed, his wife is sitting with him, and Dr. Turner walks in wearing a lab jacket and looking obviously like a doctor.

Dr.Turner asks "How are you John?"

John replies, "I'm good, ready to go home, when do you want me to take this catheter out?"

Dr. Turner asks "You don't want me to do it?"

John says, "No, I can do it. I'll email you about how I am doing. How many days do I have to wear it? I'd rather not come back to Atlanta."

Dr. Turner says "Take it out on post-op day six."

John says, "Perfect, I'm giving a party on Saturday for the operating room, and I'd rather be in diapers than wearing a catheter."

Dr. Turner frowns, as does the wife in the background.

Dr. Turner says, "Saturday, this Saturday, tomorrow?"

John says, "No, not this Saturday, next Saturday."

Dr. Turner says, "I don't know that you'll be up for that, but I guess we will just have to see how you do."

John says, "Thanks again for what you did for me."

Scene eight

It is the day of the party; John is trying to figure out which pair of shorts will least show the effect of the diapers underneath, looking at himself in various poses and shorts in the mirror adjacent to the kitchen, and is concerned about the diapers filling up too fast if he drinks beer and how he will be able to change the diapers with so many people around.

His wife asks, "When are you going to the party?"

John replies, "In a few minutes. I'm trying to figure out this diaper thing, I think what I need to do is have on a pair of diapers and then inside that a liner of some sort. That way I can discard the liner when it fills up with urine and replace it without taking off my shorts. Can you tell that I have diapers on now?"

John motions to his pelvic area and turns this way and that and looks at himself as his wife looks on. The wife blatantly looks at her husband's crotch area in an exaggerated fashion as if unabashedly making a point to look. She then shakes her head as if the whole process is silly.

She says "Well, you could if you were just looking there, but I don't think people will be doing that."

John says, "I think I'm going to stop by the pharmacy and get a new supply of diapers and check out the liners; I need a system that will allow me to participate in this party and that will also work for my surgeries Tuesday. I'll see you there."

John walks out the kitchen door. *(If possible the audio over-emphasizes the crinkling sound of the plastic in his diapers.)*

Scene nine

John is in a pharmacy standing under a sign that says "incontinence aids," and he has two varieties of diapers that he is looking back and forth at as well as the other products on the shelf, comparing prices. The camera is zooming in on the brands, the particulars of each diaper and the prices. One of the products is the store brand and is "two-for-one with the Rite Aid discount card" You get the sense that John is over-thinking the process of which one to get and that he is conscientious of and embarrassed by the fact that he is in a section of the pharmacy for incontinence aids. He begins to wonder if he is being noticed or watched and if maybe someone he knows will happen to come into the store.

An attractive younger girl approaches and asks, "May I help you sir?"

John, appearing somewhat anxious, replies, "No thank you, just getting some things for my mother."

John now exhibits anxiety because he needs to get the diapers and pads, he wants to get the right kind to wear for the party at the best deal, but he doesn't like being in the incontinence aisle and feels the need to move on and go. He is late for his own party. He begins to talk to himself.

John to himself: "I need the least absorbent diaper with the smallest profile and something other than a plastic outside because it makes that damn crinkly sound when I walk. I then need a liner with the highest absorbency but the smallest size. I like the two-for-one Rite aid brand but I think brand name would be better. I need to go."

John gets the brand name diaper and the Rite Aid brand liner. The next shot is John at check out, wanting to hurry and not be seen with the diapers, probably making another reference that "these are for my mother-in-law." He makes a face when he is told he can only get the two-for-one diapers with the coupon at the incontinence aid aisle, and he has to go back to get the coupon, further embarrassing and delaying him.

The camera follows him to his truck, with a dog in it, where he rips into the liners and notices that the back of the liner is a firm foam that bulges out when he puts it in his diaper in the parking lot of the pharmacy.

John: "Damn it, I should have gotten the liner with soft backing, this foam is going to be a problem. To hell with it, I need to get there."

John gets into the car with the camera showing on the seat all sorts of diaper paraphernalia, different brands of diapers, liners, old packaging, etc. His dog is sniffing around the seat uncomfortably close to John's crotch. He pushes the dog's nose away, only to have the dog find other "continence aid" items on the floorboard to sniff and scratch at.

Scene ten

John is at the party. It is at a lake, lots of people, music, and everyone is talking and drinking beer. You see a makeshift tiki bar with inflatable plants around it and a Corona sign. John is talking with two people, and the camera accentuates that fact that his shorts are drooping in the middle and the crotch is bulging. John doesn't notice, but the camera catches the eyes of one of the women he is talking to, and she peers at his crotch when he is looking away. She makes a face. John begins to feel that the liner in the diaper is full and now is beginning to figure out how to exchange the liner and where. The camera looks all around at possibilities. The far-away porta-potty, his truck up a drive near a small cabin, the enclosed dock, the woods above where the DJ is playing the music. He makes his way to the dock and he has to waddle because of the full liner. (Only a few of the participants know that John has had surgery and that he is wearing the diapers.) John waddles across the walkway to the dock, the swaying of the dock and the waddling because of the diapers accentuates the hilarity of the situation.

In the dock, he pretends to be checking on something, and while his head is peering out the door, he quickly slips out one liner and sticks another one in and throws the old liner behind a shelf. He walks out as if nothing had happened.

In order to have a dry, non-bulky liner, John has to discard the full ones in creative ways, in between getting another beer and speaking to many people along the way. He hides them all over the area, behind the porta- potty, in the truck, the dock, the woods, and the cabin. This is done while entertaining and answering questions about how long he's had the property, what a good idea the party was, etc. At one point, a group plants a tree in memory of a deceased operating room nurse, and John is asked to say something to dedicate the tree. John's liner is full, so is he speaking but turning this way and that to minimize what he perceives is now an obvious ballooning out of his crotch. Over the course of several hours he speaks to a lot of people and is seen walking up a hill, making his way to the porta potties, going into the woods, and doing the exchange without people noticing. They do notice that he is making trips here and there and some comment on it, but they don't know why.

(While talking to a guest) again the camera emphasizing John's crotch, his dog Chloe ambles up. At his feet, with several people looking on, she begins eating and picking apart one of the poorly

hidden liners she's found. John hurriedly gets it and throws it away.

The party ends and the incessant trips by John to various areas to hide liners all about the property is well documented. The next day, John is trying to remember where he put all the liners as he begins to collect them for disposal.

Scene eleven

John is leaving the operating room. The camera follows him to the surgeon's lounge where he gets a liner out of his locker, goes into the restroom looking around very carefully to see if anyone noticed, and puts another clean liner in and discards the old liner deep in the trash can by pulling some trash out , putting in the liner, then replacing the trash. Then he goes to the consultation area to speak to the patient's wife from the earlier scene. She is sitting with a book on her lap.

John: "Good morning, Mrs. Smith. How are you?"
"I am very well thank you, just a little tired; we've been up since five."
John: "What type of diapers did you end up getting?"
Wife: *Looking somewhat puzzled*, "Just some at the grocery store."
John: "Brand name or store brand?"
Wife: "I don't remember, just adult diapers."
John: "Well, what you want is brand name *Depends*. They are in a green plastic container and in either the incontinence aid aisle or adult diaper section of the store. You want to get the hyper-absorbent type with the option of two-way use. The sides of the diaper you want are perforated and have sticky tabs on the side that

you tear, put on, and secure without taking your pants off. The material on the side breathes, and since it is breathable and not plastic, it won't make that plastic crinkly noise when he walks. If he is in public or going to church or something, I would suggest getting a liner for the inside of the diaper, and then you can change that without changing the whole diaper. Having the diaper in addition to the liner gives you a little confidence in case the liner overflows. I don't think brand name is important in terms of the liner you choose unless you are looking for a low crotch profile or if odor and skin barrier issues are a problem. You can use some grocery store discount cards for these, particularly if they are on sale."

The wife is somewhat taken aback; she is waiting to see how her husband did with the major surgery. Throughout the diaper discussion and dialogue she is making unusual faces. John is oblivious to this and is really into the various options regarding diaper management.

She interrupts: "Dr. McHugh, how did my husband do, is he ok?"
John, as if coming out of a coma or out of a daydream and showing surprise.
"Your husband, oh he's fine. The surgery went great. He should do well."

Did I treat you fairly?

W hen I was a freshman at North Georgia College in the spring of 1974, I had this plastic football with a screw-off top that could hold about a quart of my favorite liquid. Other than the fact that it was plastic, one might never know its true function. As North Georgia College is a military school, it had strict rules prohibiting alcohol on campus, so my trick football was a big hit with my friends, particularly for sneaking alcohol into on-campus events. I had stolen the ball from my brother Bob. I don't know how he got it, and I am sure he didn't suspect me of taking it – it just "went missing."

At that time, I loved the band Atlanta Rhythm Section, and I had my own bootleg version of one of their first albums (which I had of course stolen from Rushton, my oldest brother). My favorite song on the album was titled 'Back up Against the Wall'. I played it over and over, knew all the words, and I would somehow find a line in the song to apply to any situation. It just so happened that the Atlanta Rhythm Section was to be playing at the North Georgia College gym that spring of 1974, so I got the ole football out and filled it with coke and Henry McKenna whisky, and went to the concert with my friends Keith Nowicki and Bart, who loved the Marines and whose goal in life was to be a Marine. We had all taken big sips from the football in the dorm before setting out on our walk to the gym. Everything at North Georgia was situated around a large circular "drill field," so from the dorm to the gym was only about a five-minute walk. "Fill up the football, take it to the concert," we sang on the way; passing it around both as a container and as if it were a real football. We strut into the concert with the football, everybody takes a football to concerts don't they, and sit on the floor of the gym in the first row right in front of the stage. They did not play my favorite song 'Back up Against the Wall', but I remember they ended with 'Angel'. I loved that song then, and I still do. As soon as 'Angel' stopped playing, the students just got up and started walking out without doing the usual chant for an encore after the last song. And then it dawned on me that throughout the entire concert no one danced or showed any emotion. Mostly they just sat, listened quietly, and then got up and left when it was over. That there was no encore performed made me furious; I just knew if they had been encouraged to play another song, it would have been 'Back Up Against the Wall.' That, in addition to the football elixir, prompted me to talk disparagingly about my fellow students. I made a "scene," as my mother would say, all the way from the floor of the gym, through the lobby, and on out into the walkway leading away from the gym.

The following Monday, there is a sticker on my dorm door telling me to "report to the Commandant of Cadets, ASAP." I read the note, and for the life of me, had no idea what this could be about. After my first class, I dutifully report to the Military Department. It was in a separate building where all the military classes were held, and all the teachers associated with Military Science had their offices there. I announce myself, and they usher me in to see the Commandant, the head guy of the military for North Georgia College.

"Sir, I am Private McHugh, Echo Company. You wanted to see me?"

"Yes," he said. "Did you attend the concert at the gym Saturday night past?"

"Yes, Sir, I did."

"You have been reported for Conduct Unbecoming for a Cadet. Are you aware of that?"

"No, Sir, I was not."

"It says here you used language unbecoming of a cadet while leaving the gym that night, is that correct?"

"Yes, Sir, that is probably true."

"What is your side of the story, Private McHugh?"

"Well, Sir, after the concert, all the students just got up and left. They did not applaud and demand an encore." At the time, as silly as my response must have appeared to him, I truly felt that he agreed with me, and that my actions were the appropriate response to the situation.

"Well, Mac," the Commandant pronounced slowly and deliberately, "this type of behavior cannot be tolerated, regardless of how strongly you feel about not getting to hear the encore. I am going to have to give you some demerits and two hours of walking the drill field next Sunday afternoon."

All in all, I thought the meeting went well; I had done what I was accused of, I got to meet the head guy, and I thought he liked me. I felt that he was probably tired of the strictly military type students, and that I was a refreshing change from the students he interacted with all day kissing his backside. I took the demerits and walked the drill field with pride.

Zoom ahead 25 years. I am now a board certified urologist, and I find myself sitting across from a portly man of about 70 who has been referred to me for an elevated PSA, which had raised concerns in his primary care doctor. I like this man on sight, and as is my usual custom, I ask him a little about himself before getting into his medical issues. He is reading a book about some historical military event. Despite not really liking the military side of having been a cadet, I do love history, particularly military history. I have listened to the entire Shelby Foote book on the Civil War, and it is some 80 hours long. So, I ask him about the book, and he tells me he was in the military and in fact went to West Point. I had wanted to go to West Point. In fact, I had someone who could have recommended me for it, Judge Birdsong, in LaGrange, but I felt that my eyes were too bad, and I was afraid that I could not make high enough grades there to assure my getting into medical school. I also wanted to go to the Citadel, but for the same reasons, in addition to out-of-state expenses, I went to North Georgia College instead, a "poor man's West Point." As my conversation with my patient continues, he says, "In fact, Dr. McHugh, I was the Commandant of Cadets at North Georgia College."

"Really? I went to North Georgia College '73 to '77. When were you there?"

"'71 to '75," he replies.

Then it dawns on me. "I think I had to come before you for Conduct Unbecoming for a Cadet, the spring of my freshman year, which would have been 1974."

"How about that," he says, and then quickly changes the subject back to his problem. "So what do you think about this PSA business?"

I examine his prostate and we mutually agree that a prostate biopsy is order. I remember distinctly his asking a few more questions than usual about the pain part of a biopsy. It was as if the reputation of the pain associated with the biopsy had preceded itself. He was outwardly more concerned about the potential for discomfort than the potential for the biopsy being positive for cancer.

The day arrives for the Colonel's biopsy. I enter the ultrasound room, and my nurse and I position Colonel Terrell on his left side with the legs in a cannonball position so as to facilitate the ultrasound probe and the biopsy. I put on gloves (when you see children as patients, they start to cry when they see the doctor put gloves on), and I inform Colonel Terrell I am about to begin.

"Dr. McHugh, before you start, may I ask you something?" he asks, putting his right arm in the air as if making a stopping motion and lifts his head to peer over his right shoulder to align his eyes with mine.

With the probe poised at the anal verge, I say, "Yes sir, what is it?"

"You mentioned on my last visit that when I was the Commandant at North Georgia, you had to report to me for bad conduct as a cadet."

"Yes, Sir."

"Well, before you begin, I want to know if you feel I treated you fairly?"

"Yes, sir, I do."

After a deep and noticeable sign of relief, he said, "Okay, you may begin."

Colonel Terrell's biopsy came back positive for cancer; he ultimately had external beam radiation and did well from a prostate cancer perspective. Later that year, just before Christmas, he brought me a newsletter that he sent to family members and all the people he has known throughout his military career. In it he retold the story of the Commandant coming before a former cadet who is now the urologist wielding a biopsy needle, the cadet himself having come before the Commandant for disciplinary reasons years before.

What is the definition of the ultrasound probe used to do prostate biopsies? - An instrument that has an ass at both ends.

I have good news. I have prostate cancer.

I am including this story here because it ties into my prostate cancer journey. I have been sued twice (I won both) and have been an expert witness once. I have told my wife for years that I was an expert in this and that, and she always says, "You are not an expert." I say, "I am if I want to be." When I was asked to be an "expert" for another urologist in a malpractice lawsuit, it was official. I was an expert. The plaintiff in the case had had prostate cancer. I was asked to be the expert witness in 2006, which was before I knew I had prostate cancer. It is not uncommon for medical lawsuits to take years to develop, so by the time this case came around for court, I was about a year beyond having my prostate removed. When the lawyer called to tell me the date of my deposition (a fact-finding, pre-trial questioning of the major players in a lawsuit), I told him, "I have good news. I have prostate cancer. Feel free to use the knowledge of this if you think it will help the case." I then asked, "Should I mention that I have prostate cancer to the lawyer at the deposition?" The lawyer said, "Only if he asks." The deposition was done at my office, the plaintiff's attorney never asked, and I did not mention the fact that I had prostate cancer. I felt that a jury would value my testimony much more given the fact that I had been through a little of what the patient who was suing had experienced. The date of the trial was finally set, and I began to review all the depositions in earnest. I then began to worry that if I messed up with anything I said, it could hurt the urologist I was supposed to be helping. A friend of mine, who is an attorney, had come to hear my testimony several years ago at the first of my two lawsuits. At lunch following the testimony I had asked him how he thought I did. "You talk too damn much, McHugh." I had a fear that in this case I would "talk too much," and I told the attorney that. He arranged for me to meet and be advised by a "Jury consultant", not to be told what to say, but to learn how to say it and what to emphasize in my testimony. We talked about the case in general, and I asked some questions about how he might use my prostate cancer history. "I can get pretty graphic with what I've been through if you think it would help." "Dr. McHugh, we basically have two types of expert witness: the professorial type and the type that has passion. You are the passionate type." He then adds, turning to look at the attorney, "Bill, he's good; he'll do well for you."

Something I had learned from my having been sued was that the attorneys try to make out the expert witness to be a "hired gun" who is only there to say what he is told for money. I remember my attorney asking the expert witness testifying against me how much he made an hour and how much he was paid to fly to Gainesville and back from St.Louis. The questioning went on and on so that the point was not lost on the jury. I remember my attorney leaning on the jury box as "their" expert witness explained all the money he was to make coming to our "small southern town to testify against one of our doctors." It was beautifully executed by the attorney, I remember this vividly, and I did not want that to happen to me. I told the attorney who asked me to be the expert that I planned to give the money I make to my church and I asked, "In general how much money do I make for doing this?" He gives me a broad range of a per-hour fee for the time spent reviewing the medical history and the depositions. I was not told nor did I request specifics of how much I would be paid, and I purposely did not want to receive any funds for my services before the case.

On the day of the trial, I was supposed to be "called" in the morning but it was changed at the last minute to the afternoon. "The plaintiff's attorney is going painstakingly slow," I was told. The significance of this delay was huge. I was able to review almost all of the depositions a second time, particularly the plaintiff's deposition. I found some very revealing quotes in my second review that I had not seen initially. As I had been formulating my strategy over the last few weeks before the trial, re-reviewing his deposition was invaluable. The quotes he had used in his deposition fit in nicely with what I had intended to use as an argument. I had seen them before, but seeing them after I had time to digest all the information about the case allowed me to use them in their rightful and most powerful perspective. (I viewed my role in all this not as testifying against the plaintiff, but rather, testifying that what the urologist did was within the standard of care. In other words, would I have done the same thing if I had been in the exact same situation? It is hard to criticize decisions made by another in the heat of battle.)

My heart is pounding away outside the courtroom, and I was thinking that I didn't want to mess up. I kept reminding myself: I know urology, I know prostate cancer, and I know the specifics of this case. As I waited, I began to look again at their expert witness's deposition, and I saw where he was quizzed about how much he charged for his expert services: "$250 an hour for reviewing depositions, $350 for my office deposition, and $5000 for my in-court testimony." Of course the attorney asked the questions several times in different ways in order for it to hit home with the jury, just like I remember him doing it years ago. He then asked, "Portal to portal?" The expert witness said, "Yes." Then the attorney asked, again for the benefit of the jury, "Portal to portal meaning that you are reimbursed separately for airfare, food, and accommodations, is that right?" The expert said, "Yes." I could see it in my mind's eye the attorney leaning on the jury box rail and looking back and forth between the expert and the jury as if to say, "That's a bunch of money, makes you wonder if he is an expert just for the pay." I was really getting into this particular deposition and enjoying the gamesmanship of the attorney when I heard someone announce, "Dr. McHugh, they are ready for you now."

No sooner did I sit down and do the pledge stuff, worrying that I'd use the wrong hand, the plaintiff's attorney wants to know if I had been paid anything and how much was I going to charge. "I don't know what I will be charging." He says, "You mean to tell me you don't know what you will charge?" "Yes, sir, I don't know, I have never done this before." Once I got over the dry mouth (and I mean parched dry) and the nervousness that preceded my testimony, I was fine. It so happened that I saw the bailiff as a patient several weeks later and he commented,"Doc, I filled up your water pitcher more times than I ever had before! Man you were one thirsty doctor that day!" In fact, I enjoyed testifying, particularly when he asked me a question in which the urologic premise was wrong. On several occasions he asked a question in which the details were incorrect. I would answer but only after telling the attorney that the number of days he referred to was wrong or that "that's not the appropriate terminology for what you are wanting to express." He kept using "urinary retention," which implies that a patient cannot void at all, when what he needed to say was "obstructive voiding symptoms." I was impressed, and it gave me confidence, that he had a very bad working knowledge of urology; I may have been in "his territory" by being in a courtroom, but he was clearly in my territory regarding the subject matter of the questioning. I enjoyed testifying from that point on, correcting several of his questions and then answering them in a favorable fashion for our case by using the exact quotes from the plaintiff that I had read in his deposition just minutes before. I was disappointed that it came to an end. Things would have gone on longer had it not been for the plaintiff's lawyer acknowledging that Thursday was the night the judge went out to eat. The judge agreed and said "Why don't we wrap things up counselor."

Reflecting later that evening, although initially I thought I did alright, I began to think that maybe I had been "clever by half." What if the jury thought I was too cocky or that I talked too much? Then it dawned on me that I had not played the "prostate cancer card." I just forgot about it. I began to go over the whole testimony in my mind, answering the questions much better and throwing in something about "I wore a catheter too; I know how he feels." About this time, and with me beating myself up and telling my wife that I probably did talk too much, the phone rings. It is the urologist calling to tell me that the trial would conclude tomorrow, and he'd call me with the results. He then added, "John you were great, the way you used your hands and those quotes, where did you come up with those things?" I asked, "You don't think I talked too much? I can't believe I did not mention the fact that I have prostate cancer." "No you did fine, thanks for agreeing to do what you did; I'll call you tomorrow with the verdict." The next day he called and told me that the jury found in his favor. About a week later I received a letter from the attorney telling me that my testimony played a large role in the favorable verdict and for me to submit my bill. I email the attorney's legal assistant and again asked her for advice as to what to charge. She responded that most doctors bill around $250-$350 per hour for the time they spend on a case.

Around about this time, I had another legal issue come up regarding a business matter, and I had sent a contract to a lawyer in Atlanta to review. What the lawyer did was review the contract I sent him and then send me a bill for three hours of reviewing the contract, but he did not advise me about the contract. In other words, I guess, if I want to know what he thinks about his review, I would have to ask him about that and then get another bill for him to tell me. Then it dawned on me how I should handle my bill for being an expert witness. I needed to think like an attorney, not a doctor. After about a month of "pondering" my charges, I decided submit a bill that was the same as the other expert witness. When I sent it in I prefaced the itemized expenses with, "I have decided to charge what the guy that lost charged." I got my check a few days later, my wife and I added a little to it, and it covered my commitment to my church for that year. As my mother would say, "God works in funny ways."

John, I heard you got cancer!

A fter I found out I had cancer, I decided that I would not tell but a few people. I had no reason for feeling that way, it was what it was, and it is just how I felt about it. I wanted to be able to say, "A few months ago I had my prostate removed, and everything's fine now." There was something about the telling of my situation after the fact and with hopefully a good report that was appealing to me. In a sense this method down-played my predicament and somehow lessened the drama of it to me. So when an anesthesia colleague of mine called me about a month after my surgery to go fishing, I found myself in a quandary. I had been back working for several weeks and essentially no one at my hospital knew that I had cancer, that the prostate had been removed, or that I was wearing diapers and leg bags. My partners knew, but I told them, "If anyone finds out about this, I'd like to be the one to tell them. Please let me decide that, so keep it to yourself." They took it very seriously to honor my request. In retrospect I am very grateful to them for respecting my wishes. If you think my concern about "who does the telling" is odd, it may well be, but consider an incident that happened to me during this time. Shortly after I informed my brother Bob, who lives in Atlanta, about my cancer, he told a friend who lives in my home town of LaGrange, Georgia, who in turn told his brother. Bob's friend's brother ran into my brother Cooper in a grocery store in LaGrange and told him he was sorry about John having cancer. I had not told Cooper yet, so he calls me, disappointed and embarrassed to have found out about his brother that way from a casual friend in a grocery store. I now understand why H.I.P.P.A. (Health Information Patient Protection Act) is a big deal. Back to the story: I was in my office when my nurse said there was a phone call for me. "John, this is Tom and I was wondering if we could go fishing up at your river place this Thursday afternoon." Fishing is my passion, so someone asking me if I want to go fishing is, as my mother used to say, "Like Br'er Rabbit saying to the fox, 'Oh, please don't throw me in the briar patch.'" The little cabin that Tom mentioned is a small structure on the Chattahoochee River near the Habersham and Hall County line, an area Sidney Lanier mentions in the opening lines of his poem "The Song of the Chattahoochee": *Out of the hills of Habersham/Down the valleys of Hall...* (My mother loved this poem; my grandfather's home place was on the Chattahoochee River just south of LaGrange, Georgia.) The beauty of the place is that this area of river holds what some call Georgia's unofficial state fish, the shoal bass. "Shoalies" behave like bass in their fighting ability and tastes for food, but live in and around rocks (shoals) in moving water like trout. They are a joy to catch with a fly rod. In the cabin I have several rods that I have made and all the necessary materials and equipment to tie all the flies with which I fish. To catch a fish on a rod you built and on a fly you tied, well, "It don't get no better than that!" Tom and I had gone fishing a couple of times together on the Chattahoochee River in this area. "Sure, Tom. I am up there all the time, so it's no big deal. I'd love to go." Then I realized that at some point during the trip, it's about 30 minutes from my office, I'd need to change a diaper or expose my leg bag, depending on the collection device of choice for that day. (Something I learned while at the beach the week after my surgery was that if I am near water, I don't have to wear any protection because any wetness on my shorts or bathing suit would be assumed to be water.) I had fished about a week before in some fishing shorts without a diaper, and it worked out well. I just let it flow while I was in my kayak fishing the section of the Chattahoochee near my cabin. "Tom, I need to tell you something; I had my prostate removed about a month ago, and I am still leaking urine. At some point in our outing I'll have to either change a diaper or be wet, and I wanted you to know that now." "John, what? I had no clue. For prostate cancer?" "Yes, it went well, I am fine, it was really no big deal." My response and the information after the fact were executed just as I had envisioned. "Are you sure you want to go?" "Yes, its fine. I will just have to do some things about the leakage from time to time, I'll will just let it leak while I am in the kayak and jump in the water more often than I normally do."(We'd each have our own kayak if you are wondering if there was going to be an issue with fishing in the same kayak with an incontinent friend.) "Well O.K., where do you want to meet?" "You come to my office and we can go from there, and then your car will be on the way home coming back." We go up Highway 985 north, and take Duncan Bridge Road to get to the river. I explained as we drove about how I had gone to great lengths to continue on with things without telling people about my cancer or recent surgery. He said that he had heard nothing of it. I mentioned that I felt some people at times looked at me differently, like" they knew." (Only on one occasion had someone asked me if it were true that I had had surgery for prostate cancer. It was a female gynecologist, and when two nurses nearby quickly looked away somewhat awkwardly, she immediately asked, "Did I say something I shouldn't have?" There were people who did not know, and some who knew, and, although they would not tell me they knew, I could feel it. Some people began to treat me differently, a little nicer I thought, as if maybe they felt sorry for me. I began to be sensitive to the fact that if someone was acting nicer or more deferential to me, they must know. I did not want pity or whatever it was they were doing that was different than before, but I did like it, and it changed me. I began to be nicer as well, thinking I don't want to mess up the aura of good will that is being shown to me. I remember Bill Clinton saying of George Bush that America had the good will of the world after 9/11 and we squandered it going to war with Iraq. I don't necessarily agree with that political view, but it fit for me and it became my model; don't do something mean as a doctor or as a person and lose this thing you have going on. There are lots of times in the course of an operation for the surgeon to be mean-spirited in his tone or actions, so I was on my guard not to be "myself." I was inappropriate during a surgical case one time, and after I apologized to the circulating nurse she said, "That's O.K. Dr. McHugh, we know how you are." It was actually a learning process for me in appropriate physician social behavior, and I have retained, or at least tried to retain, some of the good habits I developed during this time.)

On the way I decided to stop at a country store to get some night crawlers. The deal on live bait is that if all else fails, it is the best thing to use to catch fish. I personally rarely use live bait, but when I take someone fishing, it is a nice fallback if no fish are being caught. We arrive at this little store that has the bait, Creekside Trading Post, which is about two miles from the river and cabin and really "off the beaten path." Tom says, "I'll go in with you to see what other tackle they have." When we go in the store, I see sitting on a stool in front of the cash register a neighbor who has a cabin near mine on the river. He lives by himself, and I imagine must have an afternoon ritual of having a coke at this store and visiting with the owner. There were several other customers in the store when Tom and I entered. I had just finished up my conversation with Tom about my previously mentioned revelations and intentions about "keeping my disease quiet," when my river neighbor sees me and yells across the expanse of the store, "Hey John, I heard you got cancer!" I turned and looked at Tom with a "Now that was funny!" look and then at my neighbor to nod. I then shifted my attention to the guy at the cash register and asked nonchalantly, "Y'all got any night crawlers?"

After the "store" episode, I slowly began to tell people in an ever-broadening circle of who I felt should know. One particular group of the "enlightened" were my patients who had prostate cancer. For many of them, I had removed their prostate and probably seen them at a previous office visit in my urine collection "contraption" without their knowledge. I would say it took about a year and half for me to begin to more liberally tell people about my prostate cancer, and it was nice to be able to do so retrospectively. My patients that were beginning the journey themselves, I felt, seemed comforted by knowing their doctor had been through what they were going through. I think I now can sense a patient's anxiety about a particular facet of the disease and address it much better.

My hesitancy in telling others about my prostate cancer and that I probably made a bigger deal out of it than necessary, reminds me of the time I informed my daughter about my first law suit. She was to be the Sugar Plum Fairy in our hometown's ballet company production of the "Nutcracker" and she and her mother were looking at ballet shoes in a magazine. "Bess, I want to tell you that I will be in court all next week for a malpractice lawsuit. One of your friends at school or maybe a teacher may mention or ask you something about it, and it could be in the paper. Daddy has not done anything wrong, it isn't like I could go to jail or anything, it is just something that happens to doctors these days, and it will be

O.K." Again, just like my aunt said of my grandfather Robert Cooper Davis, I began to feel the moistness in my eyes beginning; I hate that when it happens. Bess looks at me for a few seconds and then at her mother and says, "Mom, I think I like the pink ones better." It was probably the best thing she could have said.

Made in the USA
Lexington, KY
17 December 2014